Acute Medicine

a practical guide to the
management of medical emergencies

Acute Medicine
a practical guide to the
management of medical emergencies

David Sprigings MA MRCP
Consultant Physician, Northampton General Hospital

John Chambers MA MD MRCP
Senior Lecturer and Honorary Consultant Cardiologist,
Guy's Hospital, London
and Maidstone Hospital

Andrew Jeffrey BSc FRCPE
Consultant Physician, Northampton General Hospital

SECOND EDITION

**Blackwell
Science**

© 1990, 1995 by
Blackwell Science Ltd
Editorial Offices:
Osney Mead, Oxford OX2 0EL
25 John Street, London WC1N 2BL
23 Ainslie Place, Edinburgh EH3 6AJ
238 Main Street, Cambridge
  Massachusetts 02142, USA
54 University Street, Carlton
  Victoria 3053, Australia

Other Editorial Offices:
Arnette Blackwell SA
  1, rue de Lille, 75007 Paris
France

Blackwell Wissenschafts-Verlag GmbH
  Kurfürstendamm 57
  10707 Berlin
  Germany

  Feldgasse 13
  A-1238 Wien
  Austria

First published 1990
Reprinted 1991, 1992, 1993, 1994
Second edition 1995
Reprinted 1996

Set by Excel Typesetters, Hong Kong

Printed and bound in Great Britain
at the University Press, Cambridge

DISTRIBUTORS

  Marston Book Services Ltd
  PO Box 87
  Oxford OX2 0DT
  (*Orders*: Tel: 01865 791155
             Fax: 01865 791927
             Telex: 837515)

North America
  Blackwell Science, Inc.
  238 Main Street
  Cambridge, MA 02142
  (*Orders*: Tel: 800 215-1000
              617 876-7000
              Fax: 617 492-5263)

Australia
  Blackwell Science Pty Ltd
  54 University Street
  Carlton, Victoria 3053
  (*Orders*: Tel: 03 347-0300
             Fax: 03 349-3016)

A catalogue record for this title is available from
the British Library

ISBN 0-632-03652-4

Library of Congress
Cataloging-in-Publication Data

Sprigings, David.
  Acute medicine: a practical guide
  to the management of medical
  emergencies/David Sprigings, John
  Chambers, Andrew Jeffrey. – 2nd ed.
        p.   cm.
  Includes bibliographical references
and index.
    ISBN 0-632-03652-4
    1. Medical emergencies – Handbooks,
manuals, etc. I. Chambers, John, MD.
II. Jeffrey, Andrew.   III. Title.
[DNLM: 1. Emergencies – handbooks.
WB 39 5769a   1995]
RC86.8.568   1995
616.02'5 – dc20

Contents

Preface to the second edition

The safe and effective management of medical emergencies requires an approach very different from that described in most textbooks. *Acute Medicine* is intended to be a practical guide for the front-line doctor. For this second edition, we have revised all chapters to take account of advances in diagnosis and treatment over the past 5 years, and have added three new ones (on acute medical problems in the patient with HIV/AIDS; haemoptysis; and transient ischaemic attack).

D.C.S., J.B.C., A.A.J.
Northampton 1995

Acknowledgements

We are indebted to the following colleagues for expert criticism of sections of the manuscript of the second edition: John Birkhead, Charles Fox, Alan Ogilvie, Yaver Bashir, John Henry, Mark Wilkinson, Professor Gwyn Williams and Derrick Crook.

Section 1
Common Presentations

1 Cardiac arrest

Cardiac arrest is defined as the **sudden loss of consciousness with absent femoral or carotid pulses**. The commonest cause is **ventricular fibrillation** (VF).

Basic life support

1 **Basic life support** (Fig. 1.1) should be started in any nonventilated, unmonitored patient with cardiac arrest.
   - **In witnessed ventricular fibrillation** (monitored patient), **basic life support should be preceded by a single precordial thump followed by defibrillation (three shocks at 200 J, 200 J and 360 J).**
2 **Ventilation.**
   - Extend the neck, lift the chin and clear the mouth (by finger and suction).
   - In hospital, specialized masks and self-inflating bags (e.g. Ambu and Laerdal systems) may be available. It can be difficult to achieve adequate ventilation with these if you are inexperienced, in which case you should use an expired air ventilation mask or direct mouth-to-mouth breathing.
   - Do not attempt endotracheal intubation unless you have been trained to do so and no anaesthetist is available.
3 **Chest compression.**
   - Press on the sternum, not the ribs, and aim for compression of 5 cm at 80/min.
   - In single-person resuscitation give 15 compressions: 2 breaths. In two-person resuscitation give 5 compressions: 1 breath.

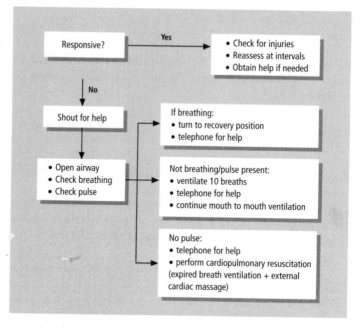

Fig. 1.1 Basic life support. From European Resuscitation Council Working Party guidelines. *BMJ* 1993; 306: 1587–93.

Advanced cardiac life support

1 The algorithms for **advanced cardiac life support** are given in Fig. 1.2. **They assume that basic life support has been initiated and is continuing**.

2 Adrenaline (1 mg IV) should be given in each cycle (i.e. every 2–3 min) to enhance basic life support, irrespective of cardiac rhythm.

3 If venous access cannot be established, adrenaline and atropine can be given via an endotracheal tube: give twice the dose used IV, diluted with isotonic saline to a volume of 10 ml.

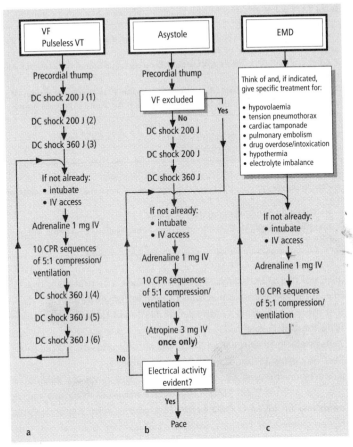

Fig. 1.2 Advanced cardiac life support: **a**, ventricular fibrillation or pulseless ventricular tachycardia; **b**, asystole; **c**, electromechanical dissociation (EMD). From European Resuscitation Council Working Party guidelines. *BMJ* 1993; 306: 1587–93.

4 Sodium bicarbonate administration should ideally be guided by arterial blood pH: if this is not known, 50 ml of 8.4% solution (50 mmol) may be given after three unsuccessful loops.

5 If plasma potassium is low (< 3.5 mmol/l): give potassium chloride

■ **Table 1.1** Cardiac arrest with hyperkalaemia (plasma potassium > 6 mmol/l)

1 Give 10 ml of calcium chloride 10% IV over 5 min. This can be repeated every 5 min up to a total dose of 40 ml
2 Correct metabolic acidosis with sodium bicarbonate 50 mmol IV (50 ml of 8.4% solution) over 10 min
3 Give dextrose 25 g (50 ml of dextrose 50%) with 10 U of soluble insulin IV over 15–30 min. This will usually reduce plasma potassium for several hours

■ **Table 1.2** Drug therapy of ventricular fibrillation or tachycardia (in conjunction with DC countershock)

• **Lignocaine:** 100 mg (5 ml of 2% solution) IV over 30 s
• **Procainamide:** 100 mg by slow IV injection every 5 min up to a total dose of 1 g
• **Amiodarone:** 150–300 mg IV over 1–2 min
• **Bretylium:** 5 mg/kg IV bolus, followed by 10 mg/kg IV after 5 min if VF persists

20 mmol (1.5 g) in 100 ml of dextrose 5% via a central vein, over 15 min. **If plasma potassium is high (> 6 mmol/l):** see Table 1.1.
6 If there is refractory ventricular fibrillation or tachycardia, consider drug therapy (Table 1.2).
7 Asystole: give adrenaline 5 mg IV if no response after three loops. Recovery after 15 min of asystole is very rare.
8 Electromechanical dissociation (EMD): the place of calcium in the management of EMD remains controversial. **Calcium should definitely be given if EMD occurs in a patient with hypocalcaemia, hyperkalaemia or calcium antagonist poisoning:** give calcium chloride 10 ml of 10% solution IV over 5 min.

Problems

When to stop resuscitation

• There is no universally applicable rule.
• In most cases resuscitation should be stopped after 30 min if there

is **refractory asystole or electromechanical dissociation**. Other rhythms may imply a potentially salvageable heart.

• Where cardiac arrest is due to **hypothermia** or **poisoning**, patients have survived neurologically intact after even longer resuscitation attempts.

• In patients without myocardial disease, do not stop resuscitation unless arterial pH and potassium are normal, and core temperature is $> 36°C$.

• Remember that adrenaline causes dilatation of pupils: this should not be used as evidence of irreversible neurological damage during or immediately after resuscitation.

What to do after successful resuscitation

1 Decide why the arrest occurred (Table 1.3). Correct low or high potassium, hypoxia and acidosis. Consider prophylactic anti-arrhythmic therapy for patients in whom arrest was due to VF/ventricular tachycardia (VT) (p. 13), bearing in mind that these drugs have a negative inotropic effect.

2 The patient should be transferred to the CCU or ITU, with ECG monitoring during transfer.

3 Mechanical ventilation should be continued for coma, severe pulmonary oedema, $Pao_2 < 9\,kPa$ (70 mmHg) (on 60% oxygen) or $Paco_2 > 6.5\,kPa$ (50 mmHg).

4 The airway should be protected until the patient is fully conscious with an intact gag and cough reflex.

■ **Table 1.3** Urgent investigation after successful resuscitation

---

- **ECG** (? acute myocardial infarction, long QT interval)
- **Chest X ray** (? pulmonary oedema, pneumothorax, rib fracture)
- **Arterial blood gases and pH**
- **Plasma potassium**
- **Blood glucose** (by stick test)

---

5 Arterial blood pressure should be maintained using inotropic/vasopressor agents if necessary (p. 40): tissue perfusion needs to be restored as quickly as possible.

6 IV lines inserted without sterile technique during the resuscitation should be changed.

2 Cardiac arrhythmias

The **haemodynamic effects** of the arrhythmia determine your approach to management.

- **Severe haemodynamic compromise** (cardiac arrest, reduced level of consciousness, severe pulmonary oedema, systolic BP < 90 mmHg): **immediate treatment**.
- **Moderate compromise** (signs of low cardiac output but systolic BP 90–110 mmHg, pulmonary oedema, angina at rest): **urgent treatment**.
- **Mild or no compromise**: you have time to decide what treatment (if any) is needed.

Tachyarrhythmias (rate > 120/min)

Severe compromise
- If there is cardiac arrest: manage along standard lines (Chapter 1).
- Record a 12-lead ECG (if possible) for later analysis.
- Apply DC countershock, starting at 200 J (p. 345).

Other patients
- There is time to make an electrocardiographic diagnosis before treatment.
- The initial classification is by the QRS width and regularity.

Broad-complex tachycardia (QRS width > 120 ms)

- The differential diagnosis is given in Table 2.1.

Regular broad-complex tachycardia

An approach to the diagnosis is summarized in Fig. 2.1: it is based on the **history**, the **12-lead ECG features** (Table 2.2), and the response to **adenosine** (Table 2.3).

■ **Table 2.1** Differential diagnosis of broad-complex tachycardia

Regular	• Ventricular tachycardia
	• SVT or atrial flutter with bundle branch block
	• Pre-excited atrial flutter (WPW)
	• Antidromic re-entrant tachycardia (WPW)
Irregular	• Atrial fibrillation or flutter with bundle branch block
	• Pre-excited atrial fibrillation (WPW)
	• Torsade de pointes

SVT, Supraventricular tachycardia; WPW, Wolff – Parkinson – White syndrome (Appendix 3).

■ **Table 2.2** ECG features of ventricular tachycardia

- Positive QRS concordance (predominant deflection of QRS complexes across the chest leads is positive) is seen only in VT. Negative QRS concordance may occur in both VT and SVT with aberrant conduction
- Marked left axis deviation (negative QRS in lead II) favours VT
- AV dissociation is diagnostic of VT (seen in around 25% of cases). There may also be 2 : 1 or 3 : 1 VA block rather than AV dissociation – also diagnostic of VT
- A fusion beat is a useful but rare clue to the diagnosis of VT (but may also occur in atrial arrhythmias with WPW (see Fig. 2.6, p. 31) and in SVT with BBB)
- In broad-complex tachycardia with a positive QRS in V1, VT is favoured by an Rsr' complex
- In broad-complex tachycardia with a negative QRS in V1, VT is favoured by a QS complex in V6

VT, Ventricular tachycardia; SVT, supraventricular tachycardia; AV, atrioventricular; WPW, Wolff – Parkinson – White syndrome; BBB, bundle branch block.

- **Remember that ventricular tachycardia (VT) is the commonest cause of a regular broad-complex tachycardia: if in doubt, treat for VT.**
- **Do not give verapamil as this may cause fatal hypotension in patients with VT.**
- Has the patient had a myocardial infarction and did the symptoms of the tachycardia start after the infarction? If the answer to both questions is yes, it is a near-certainty that the rhythm is VT.

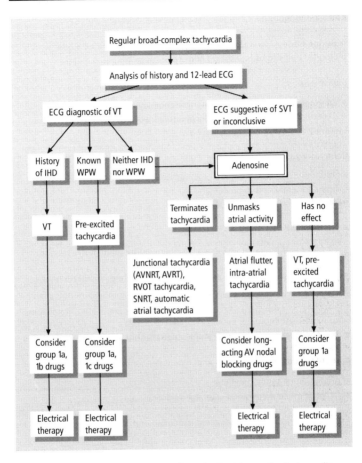

Fig. 2.1 Diagnosis and management of regular broad-complex tachycardia. AVNRT, atrioventricular nodal re-entrant tachycardia; AVRT, atrioventricular re-entrant tachycardia using an accessory pathway; RVOT, right ventricular outflow tract; SNRT, sinus node re-entrant tachycardia. From Camm AJ, Garratt CJ. *N Engl J Med* 1991; 325: 1621–9. Reproduced by permission of *The New England Journal of Medicine*.

■ **Table 2.3** Adenosine

A purine nucleoside which slows conduction through the AV node, with a biological half-life of less than 1 min when given IV

Indications

- Diagnostic test in broad- and narrow-complex tachycardia
- Treatment of SVT (re-entrant tachycardia involving the AV node or an accessory pathway)

Contraindications

- Patients with second-degree or complete AV block, or sino-atrial disease, unless a pacemaker is in place
- Asthma (a relative contraindication)

Administration

- Give as rapid bolus into a large vein, followed by saline flush, monitoring the ECG continuously
- Start with 3 mg; if no response after 2 min, give 6 mg; if still no response, give 12 mg

Adverse effects

- Transient chest discomfort, breathlessness, flushing and headache

Drug interactions

- Antagonized by theophylline
- Potentiated by dipyridamole (give half-dose)

AV, Atrioventricular; SVT, supraventricular tachycardia.

Ventricular tachycardia

Treatment

1 If haemodynamically stable, give **lignocaine 100 mg (5 ml of 2% solution) IV over 30 s.**

2 If this fails, give **procainamide 100 mg over 2 min, repeated at 5-min intervals if needed to a maximum dose of 1 g.**

3 If this also fails, use **synchronized DC countershock**. This is preferable to giving further anti-arrhythmics.

After correction of ventricular tachycardia

1 Establish the cause from the history and investigation (Table 2.4).

2 Plasma potassium should be kept in the range 4–5 mmol/l.

3 Correct hypoxia (Pao_2 should be kept > 9 kPa).

4 Correct persistent severe acidosis: if pH < 7.2 after restoration of a spontaneous output, give sodium bicarbonate 50 mmol (50 ml of 8.4% solution) IV.

5 Maintenance anti-arrhythmic therapy will usually be indicated. The following are guidelines.

  • **VT in the first 24 hours after acute myocardial infarction.** Give lignocaine by IV infusion for 12–24 hours (Table 2.5). If there are no signs of heart failure, start a beta-blocker; if there is heart failure, start an ACE-inhibitor. If VT does not recur during this period, further anti-arrhythmic therapy is not required.

  • **VT late after myocardial infarction** (usually taken arbitrarily as > 1 day) **or due to other myocardial disease**. Give lignocaine by infusion and start oral therapy: amiodarone (Table 2.6) if left ventricular function is poor; sotalol (80–160 mg 12-hourly PO) if left ventricular function is good.

■ **Table 2.4** Investigation after correction of ventricular tachycardia

  • ECG – ? myocardial infarction, long QT interval
  • Chest X-ray – ? pulmonary oedema, cardiomegaly
  • Plasma potassium
  • Plasma magnesium (if taking diuretics)
  • Cardiac enzymes (for later analysis)
  • Arterial blood gases (if there is pulmonary oedema, a reduced conscious level or evidence of sepsis)
  • Echocardiography (to assess LV function and exclude other structural heart disease)

LV, Left ventricular.

■ **Table 2.5** Lignocaine (class IB anti-arrhythmic) for treatment of ventricular tachycardia

Administration

IV, by peripheral or central vein

Loading dose

100 mg (5 ml of 2% solution) IV over 30 s

Maintenance dose (reduce by half if there is heart failure or cirrhosis)

4 mg/min for 30 min
2 mg/min for 2 hours
1 mg/min for 12–24 hours

If VT recurs, give a further bolus of 50 mg and increase the infusion rate by 1–2 mg/min

If VT recurs despite infusion at maximum dose

- Recheck plasma potassium and maintain 4–5 mmol/l
- Options are: to change to procainamide; to add amiodarone
- If these fail, seek expert advice

Toxic effects
Confusion and fits

■ **Table 2.6** Amiodarone (class III anti-arrhythmic) for treatment of ventricular tachycardia

Administration

PO or IV (preferably via a central vein to avoid thrombophlebitis)

Loading dose

IV: 300 mg (5 mg/kg) in dextrose 5% by IV infusion over 20–120 min, followed by 900 mg over 24 hours
PO: 400 mg 8-hourly for 1 week (started concurrently with IV loading), followed by 200 mg 12-hourly for 1 week

Maintenance dose

PO: 100–400 mg once daily (usually 200 mg)

Pre-excited atrial flutter and antidromic tachycardia
- See Appendix 3.

Irregular broad-complex tachycardia

Atrial fibrillation or flutter with bundle branch block
- Manage along standard lines (see p. 19 and Fig. 2.4).

Pre-excited atrial fibrillation
- See Appendix 3.

Torsade de pointes
- This is an uncommon polymorphic ventricular tachycardia characterized by QRS complexes of progressively changing amplitude and contour that seem to revolve around the isoelectric line, at a rate of 180–250/min.
- It is associated with long QT interval (usually > 500 ms) in sinus rhythm.
- The condition is usually due to therapy with anti-arrhythmic drugs which prolong the QT interval (e.g. quinidine, disopyramide, procainamide, amiodarone, sotalol), especially in patients with hypokalaemia or hypomagnesaemia.
- Treatment is with magnesium sulphate 2 g IV bolus over 2–3 min, repeated if necessary, and followed by an infusion of 2–8 mg/min.
- Use temporary pacing at 90/min (p. 332) if this is ineffective.

Narrow-complex tachycardia (QRS width < 120 ms)

- The differential diagnosis is given in Table 2.7.
- Vagotonic manoeuvres increase atrioventricular (AV) block and may reveal atrial activity. Try the Valsalva manoeuvre and carotid sinus massage (Table 2.8). If atrial waves outnumber QRS complexes, the diagnosis is atrial fibrillation, flutter or tachycardia.
- If vagotonic manoeuvres are unsuccessful, give adenosine (see Table 2.3, p. 12).

■ Table 2.7 Differential diagnosis of narrow-complex tachycardia

Arrhythmia	QRS rate (per min)	Atrial rate (per min)	Regular QRS?	Atrial activity	Effect of vagotonic manoeuvres or adenosine
Sinus tachycardia	100–200	100–200	Y	P wave precedes QRS	–
SVT	150–250	150–250	Y	Usually not seen or inverted P after QRS	++
Atrial tachycardia	100–200	120–250	Y	Abnormal shaped P wave. May outnumber QRS	+
Atrial flutter	75–175	250–350	Y	'Saw tooth' in the inferior leads/V1	+
Atrial fibrillation	<200	350–600	N	Chaotic (f waves)	+
MAT	100–130	100–130	N	P waves of three or more morphologies, irregular PP interval	–

SVT, Supraventricular tachycardia (re-entrant tachycardia involving the AV node or an accessory pathway); MAT, multifocal atrial tachycardia; – no effect or slight slowing; + slowing of ventricular rate; ++ may terminate tachycardia.

■ **Table 2.8** Carotid sinus massage

- Attach an ECG monitor (preferably with a printer)
- Check that there is no evidence of carotid artery disease (previous stroke, TIA or carotid bruit)
- The carotid sinus lies at the level of the upper border of the thyroid cartilage just below the angle of the jaw
- Massage first one side and then the other for up to 15 s, pressing over the artery with your thumb or index and middle fingers posteriorly and medially
- Stop massage if sinus rhythm supervenes or there is a ventricular pause > 2 s

TIA, Transient ischaemic attack.

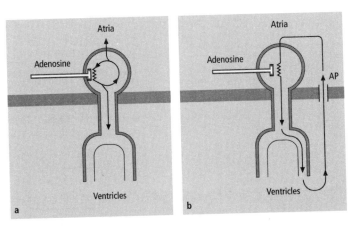

Fig. 2.2 The action of adenosine in paroxysmal supraventricular tachycardia. a, In atrioventricular nodal re-entrant tachycardia, adenosine usually blocks conduction in the slower of two pathways. b, In atrioventricular re-entrant tachycardia associated with retrograde conduction via an accessory pathway (AP), adenosine blocks antegrade conduction in the AV node. From Prys-Roberts C. *Curr Opinion Anaesthesiol* 1993; 6: 187–96.

Sinus tachycardia

- Treatment (if needed) is directed at the underlying cause.
- **Suspect atrial flutter with 2:1 AV conduction** rather than sinus tachycardia if the rate is regular at around **150/min**.

Supraventricular tachycardia

This is re-entrant tachycardia involving the AV node or an accessory pathway (Fig. 2.2).

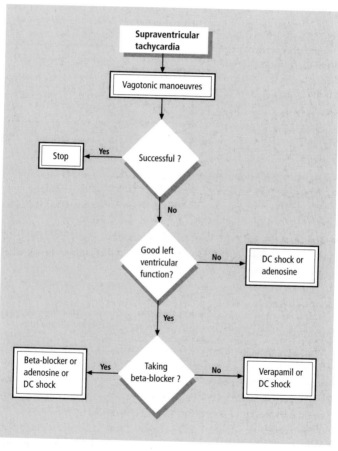

Fig. 2.3 Management of supraventricular tachycardia (AV nodal re-entrant tachycardia).

■ **Table 2.9** Drug doses in supraventricular tachycardia

Verapamil

- Start with 5 mg IV over 2 min
- If no response after 5 min, give further doses of 5 mg every 5 min to a total dose of 20 mg (10 mg in patients with ischaemic heart disease or aged > 60 years)

Adenosine (see Table 2.3, p. 12)

- Start with 3 mg IV bolus
- If no response after 2 min, give 6 mg; if still no response, give 12 mg

Beta-blocker

- Atenolol 5 mg IV **or** sotalol 20–60 mg IV

- Paroxysmal AV nodal re-entrant tachycardia is a common arrhythmia and is usually associated with a structurally normal heart.
- Management options are given in Fig. 2.3. Doses are given in Table 2.9.
- Obtain a 12-lead ECG after sinus rhythm has been restored and check that it does not show features of Wolff–Parkinson–White syndrome (Appendix 3).

Atrial tachycardia

- This is rare, but may occur as a result of digoxin toxicity (Appendix 2): therefore, withdraw digoxin.
- Check the plasma potassium and maintain at 4–5 mmol/l.
- If the arrythmia does not resolve spontaneously and digoxin toxicity is likely, consider treatment with digoxin-specific antibody fragments (see Table 2.14, p. 28). If IV anti-arrhythmic therapy is needed, use phenytoin (5 mg/kg IV over 5 min) or a beta-blocker (Table 2.9).
- If the patient is not taking digoxin and the tachycardia does not resolve spontaneously, sinus rhythm can be restored by synchronized DC countershock or a class IA anti-arrhythmic (quinidine, procainamide or disopyramide).

■ **Table 2.10** Drug doses in acute atrial fibrillation or flutter

Digoxin

Loading dose

IV: Give 0.75–1.0 mg digoxin in 50 ml of dextrose 5% or normal saline IV over 2 hours
PO: Give 0.5 mg 12-hourly for two doses, followed by 0.25 mg 12-hourly for 2 days

Maintenance dose

0.0625–0.25 mg/day. Take into account age, renal function and drug interactions

Verapamil

IV: Give 5 mg IV over 2 min. If no response after 5 min, give further doses of 5 mg every 5 min to a total dose of 20 mg (10 mg in patients with ischaemic heart disease or aged > 60 years)
PO: 40–120 mg 8-hourly

Beta-blocker

IV: Atenolol 5–10 mg by slow IV injection; sotalol 20–60 mg by slow IV injection
PO: Atenolol 25–100 mg daily; sotalol 80–160 mg 12-hourly

Amiodarone

Loading dose

IV: 300 mg (5 mg/kg) in dextrose 5% by IV infusion over 20–120 min, followed by 900 mg over 24 hours
PO: 200 mg 8-hourly for 1 week (started concurrently with IV loading), followed by 200 mg 12-hourly for 1 week

Maintenance dose

PO: 100–200 mg once daily

Flecainide (for pre-excited atrial fibrillation or flutter: see Appendix 3)

IV: 2 mg/kg to a maximum of 150 mg over 10–30 min
PO: 50–150 mg 12-hourly

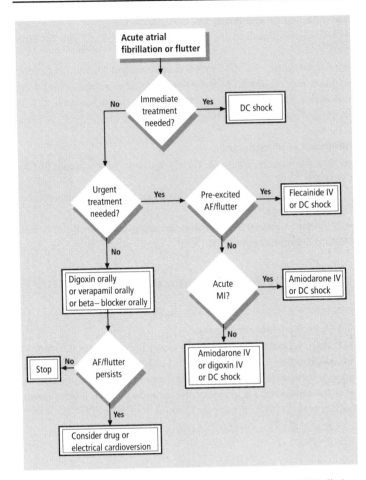

Fig. 2.4 Management of acute atrial fibrillation or flutter. AF, atrial fibrillation; MI, myocardial infarction.

Atrial fibrillation and flutter
- Management options are given in Fig. 2.4. Doses are given in Table 2.10.
- In atrial flutter, the atrial rate is usually around 300/min. In patients without intrinsic disease of the AV node or who are not taking drugs which slow conduction through the AV node, there is usually 2 : 1 AV block, giving a ventricular rate of 150/min.

Multifocal atrial tachycardia
- Most commonly occurs in elderly patients with chronic airflow limitation.
- Treatment is directed at the underlying disease and correction of hypoxia and hypercapnia.
- Consider verapamil if the ventricular rate is consistently > 110/min. DC cardioversion is ineffective.

Bradyarrhythmias (rate < 60/min)

Severe or moderate compromise
- If there is cardiac arrest: manage along standard lines (Chapter 1).
- Give **atropine 0.6 – 1.2 mg IV**, with further doses at 5-min intervals up to a total dose of 3 mg if the heart rate remains below 60/min.
- If the **bradycardia is unresponsive or recurs, put in a transvenous pacing wire** (p. 332). If necessary, whilst transferring the patient to

■ **Table 2.11** Isoprenaline infusion for bradycardia

- Add 1 mg to a 100 ml bag or 5 mg to a 500 ml bag of dextrose (5%) or saline (10 µg/ml)
- Start the infusion at 1 ml/min
- Adjust the infusion to keep the heart rate over 50/min

■ **Table 2.12** Diagnosis of bradycardia and atrioventricular block

Diagnosis	ECG features
Sinus bradycardia	Constant PR interval < 200 ms QRS regular
Junctional bradycardia	P wave absent or position constant either after, immediately before or hidden in the QRS complex
First-degree block	Constant PR interval > 200 ms
Second-degree block	
Mobitz type I (Wenckebach)	Progressively lengthening PR interval followed by dropped beat
Mobitz type II	Constant PR interval with dropped beats
Third-degree block (Complete heart block)	Relationship of P wave to QRS varies randomly P–P and R–R intervals constant but different

the screening room: either start an **isoprenaline infusion** (Table 2.11) or use an external cardiac pacing system.

Mild or no compromise
● Record a 12-lead ECG and a long rhythm strip. Look at the PR interval and the relationship between the P wave and QRS complex (Table 2.12).
● A non-conducted atrial extrasystole is often misdiagnosed as second-degree AV block.
● A regular ventricular rate < 50/min in a patient with atrial fibrillation indicates complete heart block (not 'slow AF'): always consider digoxin toxicity (Appendix 2).

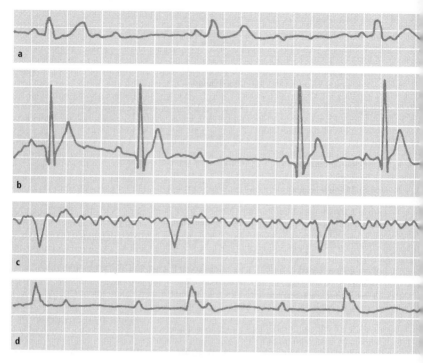

Fig. 2.5 Examples of bradycardia and atrioventricular block. **a**, Second-degree AV block (Mobitz II). **b**, Second-degree AV block (Mobitz I, Wenckebach). **c**, Complete AV block with atrial flutter. **d**, Complete AV block.

Sinus or junctional bradycardia

Related to acute myocardial infarction

This is common after inferior myocardial infarction (MI) but only needs treatment if causing hypotension, low cardiac output or ventricular escape rhythms, in which case:

- give **atropine 0.6–1.2 mg IV**, with further doses at 5-min intervals up to a total dose of 3 mg if the heart rate remains below 60/min;
- if there is little response to atropine, or frequent doses are needed, put in a temporary pacing wire.

Unrelated to myocardial infarction

• This is usually due to drugs (most commonly beta-blockers) or sino-atrial disease ('sick sinus syndrome'). Exclude hypothyroidism.

• No action is necessary if the patient is asymptomatic and the rate is > 40/min.

• If symptomatic (syncope/presyncope) or ventricular rate < 40/min, stop any drugs that may be contributing (if safe to do so), put in a temporary pacing wire and discuss permanent pacing with a cardiologist.

First-degree atrioventricular block (PR interval > 200 ms)

• This never needs treatment.

Second- and third-degree atrioventricular block

Related to acute myocardial infarction

Put in a temporary pacing wire in patients with:

• Mobitz type I second-degree AV block if there is hypotension unresponsive to atropine;

• Mobitz type II second-degree AV block;

• third-degree (complete) AV block.

Second-degree block unrelated to myocardial infarction

• Exclude digoxin toxicity (Appendix 2) or beta-blockade.

• If the patient has experienced syncope or presyncope, put in a temporary pacing wire and arrange permanent pacing.

• If asymptomatic, record a 24-hour ECG and discuss with a cardiologist whether permanent pacing is indicated.

Third-degree block unrelated to myocardial infarction

• Even in asymptomatic patients, this carries a risk of sudden death.

• Put in a temporary pacing wire if the patient has experienced syncope or presyncope, or the ventricular rate is < 40/min.

• Arrange permanent pacing.

Problems

Ventricular extrasystoles

• Ventricular extrasystoles seldom require treatment. Their significance is largely related to the underlying cardiac disease.

• Frequent ventricular extrasystoles in a patient with a central venous line may indicate that the tip of the cannula is lying against the tricuspid valve. Check the position of the tip on a chest X-ray and withdraw it if this is the case.

Reversal of beta-blockade

Beta-blockade must be reversed if contributing to pulmonary oedema, hypotension or low cardiac output.

• Give atropine and isoprenaline (dosage as above) until the heart rate is over 60/min.

• If the blood pressure remains low, start a dobutamine infusion at 10 µg/kg/min, increasing the dose as required.

• Glucagon can be combined with isoprenaline or dobutamine. Give an IV bolus of 50 µg/kg followed by an infusion of 1–5 mg/hour.

Appendix 1: suspected malfunction of permanent pacemaker

1 Check the details of the pacemaker: is it a single- or dual-chamber system, and what is the pacing mode? Contact the hospital where the system was implanted to obtain further details.

2 Obtain a 12-lead ECG, a long rhythm strip (with and without a magnet over the pulse generator (Table 2.13), and a penetrated chest X-ray (PA and lateral) for the position of the leads.

3 If these show no abnormality:

• Record a 24-hour ECG;

• Consider other causes of syncope or presyncope (Table 7.1, p. 62).

■ **Table 2.13** Diagnosis of pacemaker malfunction

Feature	Causes
No spikes*	Normal sensing Malfunction of pulse generator Spike buried in QRS complex Electromagnetic interference
Spikes without capture (failure to capture)	High threshold: • lead fracture • lead displacement • myocardial fibrosis • myocardial perforation Lead not properly connected to pulse generator Depletion of battery of pulse generator Spike in ventricular refractory period
Spikes without sensing (failure to sense)	Lead displacement Low intrinsic QRS current (i.e. not at sensing threshold)

* Placing a magnet over the pulse generator converts nearly all units to fixed rate pacing.

Appendix 2: digoxin

Therapeutic range

0.8–2.0 ng/ml (1.0–2.6 nmol/l) (blood taken > 6 hours after last dose).

Important drug interactions

Amiodarone, quinidine and verapamil increase plasma digoxin level.

Digoxin toxicity

• A clinical diagnosis, supported by measurement of plasma digoxin level. Hypokalaemia (< 3.5 mmol/l), hypomagnesaemia and hypercalcaemia predispose to toxic effects.

- Common symptoms: anorexia, nausea, vomiting, diarrhoea, headache, malaise, confusional state (in the elderly).
- Common arrhythmias: atrial tachycardia with AV block, junctional tachycardia, multiform ventricular extrasystoles.
- Toxicity is likely if plasma digoxin level is > 3.0 ng/ml (> 3.8 nmol/l), especially if there is hypokalaemia.

Management of digoxin toxicity

1 Stop digoxin.

2 Admit to the CCU for ECG monitoring.

3 Check plasma potassium and give potassium orally or IV to correct hypokalaemia.

4 Give digoxin-specific antibody fragments (Table 2.14) if significant arrhythmias or heart block occur.

5 Other therapy for arrhythmias.
- Atrial tachycardia and junctional tachycardia: see above.
- Ventricular tachycardia: lignocaine (amiodarone or phenytoin if lignocaine fails).

■ **Table 2.14** Calculation of the dose of digoxin-specific antibody fragments (Digibind, Wellcome)

Acute ingestion of unknown amount

Give 20 vials (800 mg)

Acute ingestion of known amount

Digoxin load (mg) = dose ingested (mg) × 0.8 (to take account of incomplete absorption

Number of vials of Digibind needed = digoxin load/0.6

Toxicity during chronic therapy, steady-state digoxin level not known

Give 6 vials

Toxicity during chronic therapy, steady-state digoxin level known

Number of vials of Digibind needed = plasma digoxin level (ng/ml) × body weight (kg)/100

- Second- or third-degree AV block: atropine and temporary pacing (avoid isoprenaline because of the risk of provoking ventricular arrhythmias).

NB: in digoxin toxicity, DC countershock can result in ventricular arrhythmias. Start with a 10 J shock.

Management of digoxin poisoning

1 Gastric lavage followed by activated charcoal (p. 89).
2 Check plasma potassium hourly (hyperkalaemia indicates severe toxicity and should be treated with dextrose and insulin (Table 1.1, p. 6) if > 6 mmol/l)).
3 Admit to the CCU for ECG monitoring.
4 Give digoxin-specific antibody fragments (Table 2.14) if:
   - plasma potassium is > 5 mmol/l or rising;
   - significant arrhythmias or heart block occur.

Appendix 3: Wolff–Parkinson–White syndrome

- Caused by one or more congenital muscle filaments (accessory pathways), which allow atrial impulses to reach the ventricles without conduction through the AV node.
- Characterized by a short PR interval, a widened QRS complex due to the presence of a delta wave, and a tendency to paroxysmal tachyarrhythmias (Table 2.15).
- Patients with arrhythmias associated with Wolff–Parkinson–White syndrome (WPW) should be referred to a cardiologist for consideration of electrophysiological study and catheter ablation of the accessory pathway.

Orthodromic re-entrant tachycardia

- This is the commonest arrhythmia in WPW. It is a regular narrow-complex tachycardia indistinguishable from supraventricular

■ **Table 2.15** Arrhythmias associated with Wolff – Parkinson – White syndrome

Arrhythmia	Rate (per min)	QRS width	Regularity	Management
Orthodromic AVRT (75%)*	150–250	**Narrow**	**Regular**	As for SVT (Fig. 2.3)
Antidromic AVRT (< 5%)	150–250	**Broad**	**Regular**	DC shock or flecainide
Pre-excited atrial fibrillation (20%)	May be > 250	**Broad**	**Irregular**	DC shock or flecainide
Pre-excited atrial flutter (< 5%)	May be > 250	**Broad**	**Regular or irregular**	DC shock or flecainide

Orthodromic atrioventricular re-entrant tachycardia (AVRT) is associated with activation of the ventricles via the normal conducting system and retrograde conduction over the accessory pathway (AP) (see Fig. 2.2, p. 17). Antidromic AVRT is associated with activation of the ventricles via the AP.
* Percentage of all arrhythmias associated with WPW.

tachycardia (SVT), i.e. AV nodal re-entrant tachycardia.
• Management is identical (Fig. 2.3).
• Patients presenting with SVT should have an ECG recorded when sinus rhythm is restored to identify those with WPW.

Pre-excited atrial fibrillation

• This is less common but is potentially life-threatening as very rapid atrial fibrillation (AF) (minimum interval between R waves of < 250 ms) can result in ventricular fibrillation.
• It is a broad-complex tachycardia, often misdiagnosed as VT, but distinguishable from this by the irregular RR intervals (Fig. 2.6).
• If the patient is haemodynamically stable, **flecainide** (which reduces conduction through the accessory pathway) can be used to reduce the ventricular rate and restore sinus rhythm (2 mg/kg to a maximum of 150 mg IV over 10–30 min, followed by 50–150 mg 12-hourly PO. If the patient is not stable, or you are uncertain of the diagnosis, use **DC shock. Most other anti-arrhythmics are contraindicated**, as they may

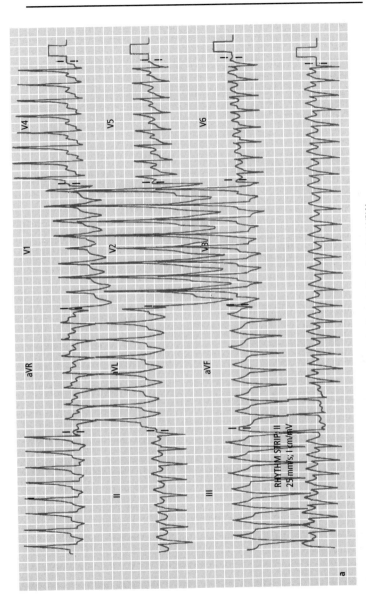

Fig. 2.6 a, Pre-excited atrial fibrillation; **b,** same patient in sinus rhythm showing WPW.

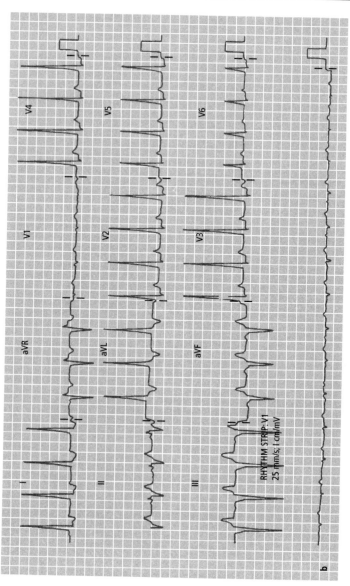

Fig. 2.6 *Continued*

shorten the refractory period of the accessory pathway and increase the ventricular rate.

Antidromic re-entrant tachycardia and pre-excited atrial flutter

- These are rare arrhythmias.
- They are broad-complex tachycardias which may be indistinguishable from VT.
- If a patient known to have WPW presents with a regular broad-complex tachycardia and is haemodynamically stable, flecainide IV may be given. In other circumstances, follow management guidelines in Fig. 2.1.

3   Hypotension

Hypotension needs urgent correction (and diagnosis of the cause (Table 3.1)) if:
- systolic BP is < 75 mmHg; or
- there are signs of low cardiac output, including confusion or drowsiness, cold skin, oliguria and metabolic acidosis.

Priorities

1 If hypovolaemia or vasodilatation are likely, lie the patient flat and elevate the foot of the bed.
2 Give oxygen. Put in a peripheral IV cannula.
3 Attach an ECG monitor. Check that breath sounds are heard over both lungs (especially if pneumothorax is possible, e.g. after recent central vein cannulation).
4 Initial management is given in Fig. 3.1.
5 Investigations needed urgently are given in Table 3.2.

Further management (Table 3.3)

1 Correct cardiac arrhythmias (Chapter 2).
- Ventricular tachycardia: synchronized DC countershock.
- AF or flutter: consider synchronized DC countershock if the ventricular rate is > 140/min (see Fig. 2.4, p. 21).
- Bradycardia unresponsive to atropine or isoprenaline: put in a temporary pacing wire.
2 Optimize the blood volume.
- Put in a central venous line – the central venous pressure (CVP) is a clue to the diagnosis (Table 3.4) and guides fluid therapy (Fig. 3.2).
- Measurement of the pulmonary artery wedge pressure (Swan–Ganz catheter, p. 323) to guide treatment should be considered if

■ **Table 3.1** Causes of hypotension

1 Cardiac pump failure	<ul><li>Arrhythmia</li><li>Acute myocardial infarction</li><li>Acute valvular lesion</li><li>Major pulmonary embolism</li><li>Cardiac tamponade</li><li>Tension pneumothorax</li></ul>
2 Hypovolaemia	<ul><li>Haemorrhage</li><li>Urinary loss</li><li>Gastrointestinal fluid loss</li><li>Cutaneous loss (e.g. burns)</li><li>Third-space sequestration (e.g. pancreatitis)</li></ul>
3 Vasodilatation	<ul><li>Sepsis</li><li>Drugs/poisoning</li><li>Anaphylaxis</li><li>Acute adrenal insufficiency</li></ul>

■ **Table 3.2** Urgent investigation in unexplained hypotension

- ECG
- Chest X-ray

- Urea, sodium and potassium
- Full blood count
- Blood glucose

- Arterial blood gases and pH

- Group and save (cross match if haemorrhage suspected)

- Culture blood and urine if suspected sepsis

- Echocardiography if:
  suspected cardiac tamponade (p. 148)
  suspected surgically correctable lesion, e.g. ventricular
    septal rupture after myocardial infarction (p. 114) or
    severe aortic or mitral regurgitation
  pulmonary oedema

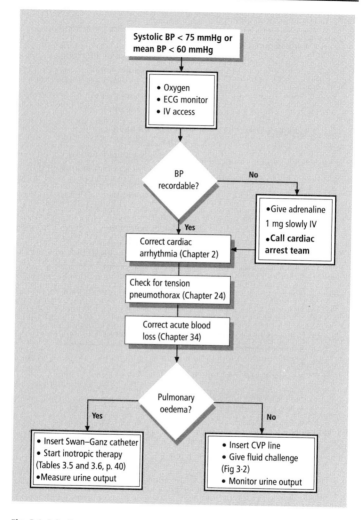

Fig. 3.1 Priority management of hypotension. CVP, Central venous pressure.

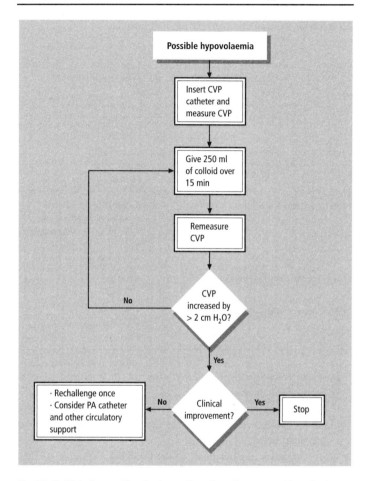

Fig. 3.2 Fluid challenge. The absolute value of CVP is a poor guide to hydration as peripheral vasoconstriction will maintain this whenever possible. Patients with sepsis may require much higher circulating volumes than normal.

■ **Table 3.3** Key points in the management of hypotension

- Correct cardiac arrhythmias
- Optimize the blood volume
- Correct hypoxia and biochemical abnormalities
- Add vasopressor/inotropic therapy
- Specific treatment of the underlying condition

■ **Table 3.4** The central venous pressure in hypotension

CVP	Causes
High (> +10 cm water)	• Biventricular failure • Pulmonary embolism • Right ventricular infarction • Cardiac tamponade • Tension pneumothorax
Low or normal with warm skin	• Sepsis • Drugs/poisoning
Low or normal with cold skin	• Hypovolaemia • Left ventricular failure • Sepsis

there is persisting hypotension despite CVP + 10 cm water or known cardiac disease (Fig. 3.3).

- Put in a urinary catheter: the urine output is an index of renal blood flow and cardiac output, and should ideally be > 30 ml/hour (> 0.5 ml/kg/hour).

3 Correct hypoxia and biochemical abnormalities.

- Maintain Pa_{O_2} > 8 kPa (60 mmHg), arterial saturation > 90%. Mechanical ventilation is indicated if Pa_{O_2} is < 8 kPa despite 60% oxygen, or Pa_{CO_2} is rising, and recovery from the underlying cause is possible.

- If arterial pH is less than 7.2, infuse 50 mmol of sodium bicarbonate (50 ml of 8.4% solution) over 15 min (severe metabolic acidosis has a negative inotropic effect and facilitates ventricular arrhythmias).

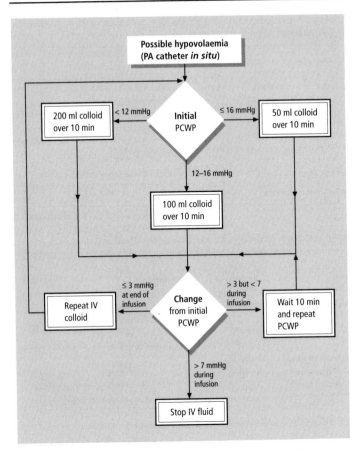

Fig. 3.3 Fluid challenge with pulmonary artery (PA) catheter *in situ*. From Bossnert LL, *et al. Drugs* 1991; 41: 857–74.

4 Consider inotropic/vasopressor therapy.

- Reverse beta-blockade (p. 26).
- If systolic BP remains < 90 mmHg despite adequate fluid therapy (CVP + 10 cm water, pulmonary artery (PA) wedge pressure 15–20 mmHg), start inotropic/vasopressor therapy (Tables 3.5 and 3.6).

■ **Table 3.5** Inotropic/vasopressor therapy for hypotension despite correction of hypovolaemia

Cause	Therapy
Cardiac pump failure	• **Dobutamine** as initial therapy • **Enoximone** can be added if needed • Consider referral for **intra-aortic balloon counterpulsation** if hypotension is due to ventricular septal rupture or acute mitral regurgitation
Septic shock	**Noradrenaline + dobutamine**
Anaphylactic shock	**Adrenaline**

■ **Table 3.6** Guide to dosage of adrenergic agonists and enoximone

Drug	Dosage (µg/kg/min)	Comment
Adrenaline	0.05	• **Beta-1 inotropic and beta-2 vasodilator effects**
	0.05–5	• **Alpha-1 vasoconstriction seen (vasopressor)**
Noradrenaline	0.05–5	
Dobutamine	5–40	
Dopamine	2.5	• **Splanchnic (renal) vasodilatation**
	5–10	• **Beta-1 mediated inotropic effect**
	10–40	• **Alpha-1 mediated vasoconstriction (vasopressor)**
Enoximone	2.5–10	• **Give loading dose of 0.5–0.75 mg/kg over 5 min first**

Adrenaline, noradrenaline and dopamine must be given via a central vein. For calculation of infusion rates see pp. 374–385.

5 **Specific treatment of the underlying condition.**
   • **Consider the causes in Table 3.1.**
   • **Hydrocortisone 200 mg IV** should be given if there is: **(a)** previous **long-term steroid treatment** (prednisolone >7.5 mg daily);

(b) suspected **primary hypoadrenalism** (preceding anorexia, nausea, vomiting and weight loss, pigmentation, low plasma sodium and raised potassium) (p. 272); **(c)** suspected **meningococcal sepsis** (young adult with fever and purpuric rash); or **(d)** suspected **anaphylaxis** (p. 296).

4 Acute chest pain

Your main aim is to confirm or exclude potentially lethal causes of pain. **If you cannot make a confident diagnosis of a minor and self-limiting disorder, admit the patient.**

Priorities

1 Check the pulse and BP, listen over the lungs and:
  • give oxygen if the patient is breathless;
  • attach an ECG monitor;
  • put in a venous cannula;
  • relieve severe pain with diamorphine 2.5–5 mg (or morphine 5–10 mg IV) plus an anti-emetic, e.g. prochlorperazine 12.5 mg IV;
  • obtain an ECG and, if the ECG is not diagnostic of acute myocardial infarction, a chest X-ray.
2 The diagnosis is often obvious from 'pattern recognition' (Table 4.1).
3 If the diagnosis is not clear within a few minutes, you need to adopt a systematic approach based on a full history and examination (Table 4.2).
4 Take another look at the ECG and chest X-ray (Table 4.3).
  • The first sign of myocardial infarction may be hyperacute peaking of the T wave, which is often overlooked. If present, relieve pain, give aspirin, heparin and nitrate (Table 13.4, p. 124) and repeat the ECG in 20–30 min.
5 Other causes of chest pain are given in Table 4.4.

Problems in diagnosis

Unstable angina vs oesophageal pain

1 Unstable angina and oesophageal pain may be indistinguishable on the history because:

■ **Table 4.1** Pattern recognition in acute chest pain

Diagnosis	Features
Myocardial infarction (p. 107)	• Pain at rest for > 30 min • ST segment elevation in at least two adjacent leads
Unstable angina (p. 122)	Pain at rest or on minimal exertion • Relief with nitrate • ST depression and/or T-wave inversion
Pulmonary embolism (p. 155)	• Pleuritic pain • Associated breathlessness • Hypoxia despite clear chest X-ray • At risk of DVT (Table 19.2, p. 153)
Aortic dissection (p. 127)	• Severe pain of **sudden** onset • Asymmetric pulses or aortic regurgitation • Abnormal chest X-ray (see Table 14.3, p. 129)
Pericarditis (p. 143)	• Central chest pain worse on inspiration, eased by sitting forward • Pericardial rub • Extensive concave ST elevation
Pneumothorax (p. 179)	• Sudden pleuritic pain • Associated breathlessness • Otherwise fit young adult • Reduced breath sounds unilaterally • Chest X-ray shows visceral pleural line with no lung markings between this line and the chest wall
Oesophageal rupture (p. 45)	• Pain following vomiting or oesophageal instrumentation • Pain worse on swallowing • Mediastinal gas • Pleural effusion

DVT, Deep-vein thrombosis.

• the distribution of myocardial and oesophageal pain may be identical (oesophageal pain may radiate to the arms);
• both may be burning or gripping in quality;

■ **Table 4.2** Clinical assessment in chest pain: points not to miss

History	• Speed of onset and duration • Exacerbating and relieving factors: ask specifically about swallowing, meals, exercise, deep breathing, and movement of the trunk and arms • Associated symptoms particularly breathlessness, haemoptysis, vomiting, neurological symptoms • Risk factors for ischaemic heart disease (smoking, positive family history, hyperlipidaemia, hypertension, diabetes), thrombo-embolism (Table 19.2, p. 153) and aortic dissection (hypertension, Marfan syndrome, pregnancy)
Examination	• Blood pressure in both arms (> 15 mmHg) difference in systolic pressure is abnormal) • All peripheral pulses • Friction rub – pleural or pericardial? • Localized chest wall tenderness? • Cardiac murmurs – especially early diastolic (aortic regurgitation as a result of dissection) • Lungs – ? pneumothorax, effusion

■ **Table 4.3** Abnormalities easily missed on the chest X-ray

- Small apical pneumothorax
- Mediastinal gas (pneumothorax or oesophageal rupture)
- Small pleural effusion (pulmonary embolism, aortic dissection or oesophageal rupture)
- Mediastinal widening (aortic dissection, oesophageal rupture)

• angina may be noticed after meals (but virtually always during exercise after meals);

• angina may be relieved transiently by belching;

2 The presence of ST depression during pain strongly favours (but is not absolutely diagnostic) of unstable angina.

3 If in doubt, admit the patient and treat for unstable angina (Chapter 13).

■ **Table 4.4** Other causes of chest pain

Common

- Oesophageal motility disorders and acid reflux
- Chest wall pain, e.g. costochondritis or fractured rib (localized tenderness)
- Cervical spondylosis (neck movement restricted and pain reproduced)
- Pleural pain (pleural rub)

Rare

- Vertebral collapse (associated 'girdle' pain)
- Herpes zoster (before the rash appears)
- Vaso-occlusive crisis of sickle-cell disease (Chapter 49)
- Intra-abdominal inflammation (e.g. cholecystitis, pancreatitis)

Chest pain related to hyperventilation

1 The diagnosis is based on:
- pain in a distribution atypical for myocardial ischaemia;
- a thoracic sighing respiratory pattern;
- exact pain reproduction by palpation, breath-holding or a hyperventilation provocation test (p. 188);
- normal ECG and chest X-ray with no hypoxia or acidosis on arterial blood gas analysis (if present, consider pulmonary embolism (p. 155) or diabetic ketoacidosis (p. 253).
3 Further management is given in Chapter 26.

Appendix 1: oesophageal rupture

Consider the diagnosis if the patient has severe chest or epigastric pain, worse on swallowing, after:

- **oesophageal instrumentation**, particularly dilatation of a stricture;
or
- **vomiting** (spontaneous rupture – Boerhaave's syndrome); (an

oesophageal tear which is not full thickness may present with bleeding (Mallory–Weiss syndrome, p. 229)).

Management

1 Obtain a chest X-ray (preferably with a lateral film as well) and look for:
- **mediastinal gas** (a crescentic radiolucent zone – may be retrocardiac or along the right cardiac border);
- **pleural effusion** (blood, gastrointestinal contents or the digestion of mediastinal pleura);
- **widened mediastinum** (haematoma).

2 If the working diagnosis is oesophageal rupture:
- give IV fluids (no oral fluids or food);
- start antibiotic therapy against Gram-negative rods and enterococci with ampicillin 500 mg 6-hourly IV, plus gentamicin IV (p. 84), plus metronidazole 500 mg 8-hourly IV.
- Discuss further investigation and management with a gastroenterologist. A large tear or continued bleeding may require surgical repair. Small tears following oesophageal instrumentation often heal spontaneously.

5   Acute breathlessness

Priorities

1 Make a rapid clinical assessment of the patient (Table 5.1).
  - Give oxygen 35–60% (or 28% if suspected chronic airflow limitation).
  - Attach an ECG monitor.

2 If there are signs of a **pneumothorax with impending cardiac arrest** insert a wide-bore needle into the second intercostal space in the midclavicular line.

3 If there is **wheeze**, give nebulized salbutamol 5 mg from the nebule or as 1 mg of nebulizer solution diluted in 2 ml of normal saline.
  - If the patient is hypoxic, but does not have chronic airflow limitation, the nebulizer should be driven with oxygen: check the necessary flow rate on the nebulizer packaging.
  - If the patient has chronic airflow limitation with known or potential carbon dioxide retention, use air as the driving gas.

4 **If there is severe pulmonary oedema** (the patient is exhaling froth):
  - correct arrhythmias;
  - give **diamorphine** 2.5–5.0 mg (or morphine 5.0–10.0 mg) by slow IV injection; **frusemide** 40–80 mg IV; **and if systolic BP is > 100 mmHg give (a), nitrate by IV infusion** (e.g. isosorbide dinitrate 2 mg/hour, increasing by 2 mg/hour every 15–30 min until breathlessness is relieved or systolic BP falls below 100 mmHg or to a maximum of 10 mg/hour), **or (b) buccal administration** (glyceryl trinitrate buccal tablet, 5 mg).

5 **Investigations required** urgently are given in Table 5.2.

6 **You should now be able to make a working diagnosis** (Table 5.3). Further management of specific problems is given in Section 2.

■ **Table 5.1** Clinical assessment of the breathless patient

History

- Preceding chest pain or palpitation?
- Increase in volume or change in colour of sputum?
- Associated wheeze?
- Past history of airways or cardiac disease?
- Risk factors for DVT (Table 19.2, p. 153)?
- Usual exercise capacity?

Examination

- Stridor?
- BP (check for pulsus paradoxus, Table 18.1, p. 149)
- JVP – raised in pulmonary embolism, cardiac tamponade and right ventricular failure (Table 3.4, p. 38)
- Heart – valvular lesion or ventricular septal rupture?
- Lungs – listen over the lung apices and laterally
- Legs – evidence of DVT or oedema?
- Sacral oedema?
- Temperature

DVT, Deep-vein thrombosis; JVP, jugular venous pressure.

■ **Table 5.2** Urgent investigation in acute breathlessness

- **Chest X-ray**
- **Arterial blood gases and pH**
- **ECG** – except in patients under the age of 40 with pneumothorax or acute asthma
- **Peak flow before and after bronchodilators** if there is wheeze or chest X-ray shows overexpanded lung fields
- **Echocardiogram** for:
  suspected cardiac tamponade
  suspected major pulmonary embolism
  possible surgically correctable cause of pulmonary oedema (e.g. ventricular
    septal rupture, severe aortic stenosis)

■ **Table 5.3** Features pointing to a diagnosis in the breathless patient

Diagnosis	Features
Asthma (p. 160)	• Wheeze with reduced peak flow rate • Previous similar episodes responding to bronchodilator therapy • Diurnal and seasonal variation in symptoms • Symptoms provoked by exercise or allergen exposure
Pulmonary oedema (p. 136)	• Cardiac disease • Bilateral interstitial or alveolar shadowing on chest X-ray
Pneumonia (p. 173)	• Fever • Cough, pleuritic chest pain • Alveolar shadowing on chest X-ray
Acute exacerbation of chronic airflow limitation (p. 166)	• Increase in sputum volume or the development of purulent sputum • Previous chronic bronchitis: sputum production daily for 3 months of the year, for 2 or more consecutive years
Pulmonary embolism (p. 155)	• Pleuritic pain, haemoptysis • Hypoxia despite clear chest X-ray • At risk of DVT (p. 153) (**NB**: signs of DVT commonly absent)
Cardiac tamponade (p. 148)	• Raised JVP • Pulsus paradoxus > 20 mmHg • Enlarged cardiac silhouette • Known carcinoma of the bronchus or breast
Laryngeal obstruction	• History of smoke inhalation or the ingestion of corrosives • Palatal or tongue oedema • Anaphylaxis (p. 296)
Tracheobronchial obstruction	• Stridor (inspiratory noise) or monophonic wheeze (expiratory 'squeak') • Known carcinoma of the bronchus • History of inhaled foreign body • $Pa\text{co}_2 > 5$ kPa (40 mmHg) (in the absence of chronic airflow limitation) • Breathlessness unresponsive to bronchodilators

Continued on p. 50

■ **Table 5.3** *(Continued)*

Diagnosis	Features
Large pleural effusion	• Distinguished from pulmonary consolidation on chest X-ray by: shadowing higher laterally than medially shadowing does not conform to that of a lobe or segment no air bronchogram trachea and mediastinum pushed to opposite side

DVT, Deep-vein thrombosis; JVP, jugular venous pressure.

Problems

Breathlessness with a normal chest X-ray

• The history and arterial blood gases (Table 5.4) give the clue.

■ **Table 5.4** Arterial blood gases in breathlessness with a normal chest X-ray

	Pa_{O_2}	Pa_{CO_2}	pH_a*
Pulmonary embolism (p. 155)	Normal/low	Low	High
Preradiological pneumonia†	Low	Low	High
Acute asthma (p. 160)	Normal/low	Low	High
Sepsis (p. 78)	Normal/low	Low	High
Metabolic acidosis (p. 398)	Normal	Low	Low
Hyperventilation without organic disease (p. 186)	High/normal	Low	High

* Respiratory alkalosis may be offset by a metabolic acidosis (Fig. 63.1, p. 399) thus allowing identification of mixed acid–base disturbances.
† Most commonly due to viruses or *Pneumocystis carinii* (p. 284).

Infection vs pulmonary oedema

Differentiation may occasionally be difficult because:

• wheeze may occur in both;

• pulmonary oedema may sometimes be localized and when severe (alveolar) it may produce an air-bronchogram;

• the radiological signs of pulmonary oedema are modified by the presence of lung disease, e.g. chronic airflow limitation;

• the two may coexist.

Management

1 Recheck the history, signs and ECG.

2 Nebulized salbutamol or aminophylline IV can be used as initial treatment for wheeze whichever the cause.

3 If fever and productive cough are absent and the white-cell count is $< 15 \times 109/l$, give frusemide and assess the response. Repeat the chest X-ray the following day.

4 If the diagnosis remains unclear, arrange echocardiography or pulmonary artery catheterization.

Tamponade vs cardiomyopathy

1 Confusion may occur because both cause:
  • enlargement of the cardiac shadow on the chest X-ray;
  • a raised JVP.

2 Points in favour of tamponade are:
  • known malignant disease, especially carcinoma of the bronchus or breast;
  • pulsus paradoxus > 20 mmHg;
  • absence of pulmonary oedema;
  • ECG normal, apart from sinus tachycardia and reduced voltages;
  • straight left-heart border on chest X-ray.

Management

1 Echocardiography should be obtained urgently.

2 Never attempt pericardiocentesis (p. 341) without echocardiographic confirmation of a pericardial effusion, except where there is imminent cardiac arrest.

Upper airways obstruction

Clues to the diagnosis are given in Table 5.3.

Management

1 Discuss management with an ENT surgeon or a chest physician.

2 If there is stridor with the strong suspicion of a carcinoma of the bronchus, start dexamethasone 4 mg 8-hourly IV.

6   The unconscious patient

- **Your first aim is to maintain adequate respiration and circulation to prevent neurological damage.**
- Poisoning is the commonest cause of non-traumatic coma in young adults.

Priorities

1 Clear the airway and give oxygen. If there is no femoral or carotid pulse, follow the guidelines for resuscitation (Chapter 1).
- Remove false teeth if loose and aspirate the pharynx, larynx and trachea with a suction catheter.
- Insert an airway and give 60% oxygen by mask: if the patient is not breathing, ventilate with an Ambubag.
- If there is no reflex response (gagging or coughing) to the suction catheter, a cuffed endotracheal tube should be inserted, preferably by an anaesthetist (Table 6.1).
- Attach an ECG monitor.
- Put in a peripheral IV cannula.

2 Check blood glucose immediately by stick test. If blood glucose is <5 mmol/1, give dextrose 25 g IV (50 ml of dextrose 50% solution) via a large vein. In chronic alcoholics there is a remote risk of precipitating Wernicke's encephalopathy by a glucose load; prevent this by giving thiamine 100 mg IV before or shortly after the dextrose.

3 Check the BP and respiratory rate and listen over both lung bases.
- If the respiratory rate is less than 10/min, if the pupils are pinpoint or there is other reason to suspect narcotic poisoning, give **naloxone** (Table 6.2).
- If systolic BP is <80 mmHg (despite correction of arrhythmias) give adrenaline 0.5–1 mg IV (5–10 ml of 1 in 10 000). If systolic BP is 80–100 mmHg, and there are no signs of pulmonary oedema, give IV fluid (saline or colloid) 500 ml over 30 min, with further fluid if

■ **Table 6.1** Indications for intubation/ventilation of the unconscious patient

Clinical	• Coma due to cardiorespiratory arrest • Respiratory rate < 8/min* • No gag reflex • To protect the airway before gastric lavage (if gag/cough reflex severely depressed)
Arterial gases	• Pao_2 < 8 kPa (60 mmHg) breathing 60% oxygen • $Paco_2$ > 7.3 (55 mmHg)*

* Give naloxone if narcotic poisoning suspected (see Table 6.2).

■ **Table 6.2** Naloxone: selective opiate antagonist

1 Naloxone should be given if:
  • respiratory rate is < 10/min
  • pupils are pinpoint
  • narcotic poisoning is suspected
2 Give up to four doses of 800 µg IV every 2–3 min until the respiratory rate is around 15/min
3 If there is a response, start an IV infusion: add 2 mg to 500 ml dextrose 5% or saline (4 µg/ml) and titrate against the respiratory rate and conscious level. The plasma half-life of naloxone is 1 hour: shorter than that of most narcotics
4 If there is no response narcotic poisoning is excluded

required guided by measurement of central venous pressure (CVP) (Table 3.2, p. 37).

4 Check arterial blood gases and pH. Monitor oxygen saturation by pulse oximetry.

  • Increase inspired oxygen concentration if Pao_2 is < 8 kPa (60 mmHg) − Sao_2 < 90%.

  • If $Paco_2$ is > 7.3 kPa (55 mmHg), consider intubation and ventilation: discuss this with an anaesthetist.

  • A low $Paco_2$ is an important clue to several causes of coma (Table 6.3).

5 If coma is a complication of the therapeutic use of benzodiazepine in hospital, flumazenil (a selective benzodiazepine antagonist) may

■ **Table 6.3** Causes of coma plus hyperventilation

- Diabetic ketoacidosis (p. 253)*
- Liver failure (p. 231)*
- Renal failure (p. 238)*
- Bacterial meningitis (p. 204)
- Cerebral malaria (Table 50.4, p. 307)
- Poisoning with aspirin, carbon monoxide, ethanol, ethylene glycol, methanol, paracetamol or tricyclics (p. 86)*
- Stroke complicated by pneumonia or pulmonary oedema
- Brainstem stroke

* Associated with a metabolic acidosis.

be given (200 µg IV over 15 s; if needed, further doses of 100 µg can be given at 1-min intervals up to a total dose of 1 mg). Flumazenil should not be given to other patients because of the risk of precipitating fits if there is mixed poisoning with benzodiazepines and tricyclics.

Further management

At this stage you should obtain a full history and perform a systematic examination. Your further management depends on the neurological signs (Table 6.4 and Fig. 6.1).

The patient can now be placed in one of four groups

1 Signs of head injury (with or without focal neurological signs).
- An intracranial haematoma must be excluded.
- Check for injury to other bones and organs.
- Correct hypotension (systolic BP < 100 mmHg) with IV fluid or blood, guided by measurement of central venous pressure (CVP).
- Arrange skull, cervical spine and chest X-rays and urgent computed tomography (CT) of the head.
- Discuss further management with a neurosurgeon.

■ **Table 6.4** Neurological examination of the unconscious patient

1 Document the level of consciousness in objective terms (see Glasgow Coma Scale **Appendix 1**)

2 Examine for signs of head injury (e.g. scalp laceration, bruising, blood at external auditory meatus or from nose)

3 If there are signs of head injury, assume additional cervical spine injury until proven otherwise: the neck must be immobilized in a collar and X-rayed before you test neck stiffness and the oculocephalic responses

4 Test for neck stiffness

5 Record the size of pupils and their response to bright light

6 Test the oculocephalic response. This is a simple but important test of an intact brainstem. Rotate the head to left and right. In an unconscious patient with an intact brainstem both eyes rotate counter to movement of the head

7 Examine the limbs: tone, response to painful stimuli (nailbed pressure), tendon reflexes and plantar responses

8 Examine the fundi

■ **Table 6.5** Causes of coma with neck stiffness

- Bacterial meningitis (p. 204)
- Encephalitis (p. 210)
- Subarachnoid haemorrhage (p. 200)
- Cerebral or cerebellar haemorrhage (p. 189) with extension into the subarachnoid space
- Cerebral malaria (p. 307)

NB: In any of these conditions, neck stiffness may be lost with increasing coma.

2 Neck stiffness (with or without focal neurological signs) (Table 6.5).

- If the clinical features suggest bacterial meningitis, take blood for culture and start antibiotic therapy (p. 204).
- Malaria must be excluded in patients who have recently travelled to or through an endemic area.
- Arrange urgent CT scan.

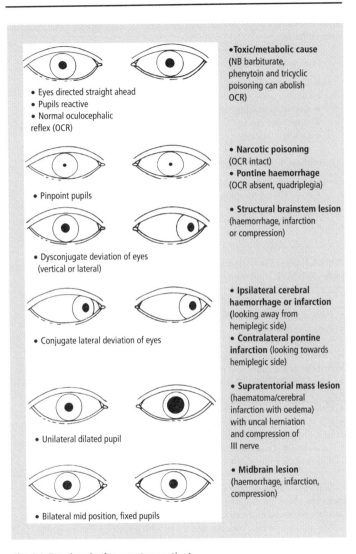

- Eyes directed straight ahead
- Pupils reactive
- Normal oculocephalic reflex (OCR)

- Pinpoint pupils

- Dysconjugate deviation of eyes (vertical or lateral)

- Conjugate lateral deviation of eyes

- Unilateral dilated pupil

- Bilateral mid position, fixed pupils

•**Toxic/metabolic cause** (NB barbiturate, phenytoin and tricyclic poisoning can abolish OCR)

- **Narcotic poisoning** (OCR intact)
- **Pontine haemorrhage** (OCR absent, quadriplegia)

- **Structural brainstem lesion** (haemorrhage, infarction or compression)

- **Ipsilateral cerebral haemorrhage or infarction** (looking away from hemiplegic side)
- **Contralateral pontine infarction** (looking towards hemiplegic side)

- **Supratentorial mass lesion** (haematoma/cerebral infarction with oedema) with uncal herniation and compression of III nerve

- **Midbrain lesion** (haemorrhage, infarction, compression)

Fig. 6.1 Eye signs in the comatose patient.

■ **Table 6.6** Causes of coma with focal neurological signs but no head injury or neck stiffness

---

With brainstem signs (deviation of the eyes or abnormal pupils)

- Brainstem compression due to large intracerebral haemorrhage or infarction with oedema
- Brainstem stroke
- Cerebellar stroke
- Cerebral malaria

Without brainstem signs

- Hypoglycaemia (in some cases)
- Liver failure (in some cases)
- Cerebral malaria

■ **Table 6.7** Urgent investigation of the comatose patient without head injury, neck stiffness or focal neurological signs

---

- Blood glucose
- Urea, sodium and potassium (? hypo- or hypernatraemia, renal failure)
- Plasma osmolality*
- Full blood count
- Prothrombin time if suspected liver failure
- Arterial blood gases and pH
- Gastric lavage (p. 91) if poisoning suspected or coma remains unexplained
- Chest X-ray
- Blood culture if temperature < 36°C or > 37.5°C
- ECG if there is hypotension, coexistent heart disease or suspected ingestion of cardiotoxic drugs (anti-arrhythmics, tricyclic antidepressants)
- **If poisoning is suspected:** save serum (10 ml), urine (50 ml) and vomit or gastric aspirate (50 ml) at 4°C for subsequent analysis

---

* The normal range of plasma osmolality is 280–300 mosmol/kg. If the measured plasma osmolality (by freezing-point-depression method) exceeds calculated osmolality (from the formula [2(Na + K) + urea + glucose]) by 10 mosmol/kg or more, consider poisoning with ethanol, ethylene glycol, isopropyl alcohol or methanol.

3 Focal neurological signs but no head injury or neck stiffness (Table 6.6).

- Exclude hypoglycaemia.
- The likely diagnosis is a stroke (p. 189).
- Arrange urgent CT if the diagnosis is unclear, or there is the possibility of an intracranial haematoma or obstructive hydrocephalus (see Table 27.2, p. 190).

4 No head injury, neck stiffness or focal neurological signs.

- The likely diagnosis is poisoning with psychotropic drugs or alcohol intoxication, but other metabolic causes must be excluded.
- Urgent investigation is given in Table 6.7.

Appendix 1: Glasgow Coma Scale

Eye opening	Score
None – the eyes remain closed	1
To pain – the eyes open in response to a painful stimulus applied to the trunk or a limb (a painful stimulus to the head usually provokes closing of the eyes)	2
To voice	3
Spontaneous – the eyes are open with blinking	4

Verbal response	Score
None – no sound whatsoever is produced	1
Incomprehensible – mutters or groans only	2
Inappropriate – intelligible but isolated words	3
Confused speech	4
Oriented speech	5

Motor response*	Score
None	1
Extensor response	2
Abnormal flexor response	3
Withdrawal	4
Localizing – uses limb to locate or resist the painful stimulus	5
Voluntary – obeys commands	6

Total score	3–15

* To assess the motor response, ask the patient to move the limb. If there is no response, apply firm pressure to the nailbed. Test and record for each of the limbs. Test for a localizing response by pressure on the supra-orbital notch or sternal rub. For the purpose of assessment of conscious level, the best motor response is taken. Differences between the limbs will be important in identifying any focal neurological lesion.

Reference:
Teasdale G, Jennett B. Assessment of impaired consciousness and coma: a practical scale. *Lancet* 1974; 2: 81–4.

7 Transient loss of consciousness

Your aim is to distinguish the more common benign causes from others that require specific treatment (Table 7.1).

Priorities

1 Was it syncope or a fit? Distinguishing between the two requires a **detailed history** (Table 7.2), taken from the patient and any eye-witnesses. Features that differentiate syncope from a fit are summarized in Table 7.3. A tonic–clonic fit may occasionally occur in cardiac syncope.

2 The **examination** (Table 7.4) is directed at excluding structural heart disease or residual neurological signs. **Initial investigation** is given in Table 7.5.

Further management

1 Admit or discharge? Patients with benign causes of syncope and no significant abnormalities on clinical examination or ECG do not need admission.

2 When is temporary pacing indicated?
- Second-degree or complete atrioventricular (AV) block.
- Sinus pauses > 3 s.
- Sinus bradycardia < 40/min unresponsive to atropine.
- Failure of permanent pacemaker system (p. 26).

3 Who should be monitored on the CCU?
- Patients with evidence of conducting system disease but without absolute indications for temporary pacing: **(a)** sinus brady-cardia, not due to beta-blockade; **(b)** sinus pauses of 2–3 s; **(c)** left bundle branch block.
- Patients at risk of ventricular tachycardia (Table 7.6).

4 In the absence of features pointing to an alternative cause, a

■ **Table 7.1** Causes of transient loss of consciousness

Common	Less common
Benign	**Cardiovascular**
Vasovagal syncope	Neurocardiogenic syncope
Micturition/cough/defaecation syncope*	Aortic stenosis
Panic disorder	Pulmonary embolism
Primary hyperventilation	Aortic dissection
	Pacemaker malfunction
	Carotid sinus hypersensitivity
Cardiovascular	Pulmonary hypertension
Arrhythmias	
Postural hypotension	**Neurological**
	Subarachnoid haemorrhage
Neurological	Vertebrobasilar transient ischaemic attack
Major fit	Subclavian steal syndrome
Others	**Others**
Hypoglycaemia	Rapid haemorrhage

* Micturition/cough/defaecation syncope: syncope occurring in these circumstances without another cause apparent on examination or ECG.

cardiac arrhythmia is the commonest cause. Clinical features and abnormalities on the resting ECG may point to a specific diagnosis (Table 7.6).

• Arrange ambulatory ECG monitoring.

• Test for carotid sinus hypersensitivity. This is performed with the patient lying down. Put in a venous cannula and draw up atropine in case prolonged asystole occurs. Attach an ECG monitor. Check the BP. Perform carotid sinus massage for 5 s (Table 2.8, p. 17) whilst recording a rhythm strip. An abnormal response is defined by a sinus pause > 3 s or a drop in systolic BP > 50 mmHg. If these occur, discuss with a cardiologist whether pacemaker implantation is indicated.

■ **Table 7.2** Was it syncope or a fit?

Background

- Any previous similar attacks
- Previous significant head injury (skull fracture or loss of consciousness)
- Birth injury, febrile convulsions in childhood, meningitis or encephalitis
- Family history of epilepsy
- Cardiac disease especially previous myocardial infarction (at risk of VT)
- Drug therapy
- Alcohol or substance abuse
- Sleep deprivation

Before the attack

- Prodromal symptoms – were these cardiovascular (e.g. dizziness, palpitation, chest pain) or focal neurological symptoms (aura)?
- Circumstances, e.g. exercising, standing, sitting or lying, sleeping
- Precipitants, e.g. coughing, micturition, head-turning

The attack

- Were there any focal neurological features at the onset: sustained deviation of the head or eyes, or unilateral jerking of the limbs?
- Was there a cry (may occur in tonic phase of fit)?
- Duration of fit
- Facial colour change
- Abnormal pulse (must be assessed in relation to the reliability of the witness)
- Associated tongue biting
- Urinary incontinence
- Any injury

After the attack

- Immediately well or delayed recovery with confusion or headache?

VT, Ventricular tachycardia.

Feature	Syncope	Fit
Occurrence when sitting or lying	Uncommon	Common
Occurrence during sleep	Uncommon	Common
Aura or warning: • duration • features	Long Dizziness, sweating, palpitation, nausea	Short Focal CNS symptoms, automatisms, hallucinations
Pallor at onset	Common	Uncommon
Tonic–clonic movements	Uncommon	Characteristic
Tongue-biting	Uncommon	Common
Incontinence	Uncommon	Common
Injury	Uncommon	Common
Postictal confusion or headache	Uncommon	Common
Postictal paresis	Never	Sometimes (Todd's paresis)

Reproduced from Schneiderman J. The first fit. *Med Int* 1992; 99: 4128 by kind permission of the Medicine Group (Journals) Ltd.

■ Table 7.4 Points not to be missed on examination

- Systolic BP sitting or lying and after 2 min standing (fall > 20 mmHg abnormal, note if symptomatic or not)
- Pulses – asymmetry, bruits
- JVP (if raised, consider pulmonary embolism or cardiac tamponade)
- Heart murmurs (aortic stenosis and hypertrophic cardiomyopathy may cause exertional syncope)
- Conscious level (confirm fully orientated)
- Neck mobility – does neck movement induce dizziness? Is there neck stiffness?
- Abnormal neurological signs?

■ **Table 7.5** Initial investigation after syncope

ECG in all patients

- Atrioventricular block or bundle branch block?
- Evidence of sino-atrial disease (see Table 7.6)?
- Signs of infarction?
- Left ventricular hypertrophy? If so, check again for aortic stenosis
- Wolff–Parkinson–White syndrome? (PR interval < 0.12 s, delta wave, may give pseudo-infarct pattern; p. 29)
- Long QT interval?

If there is postural hypotension

- Urea, sodium and potassium
- Full blood count

Cause uncertain

- Urea, sodium and potassium
- Full blood count
- Blood glucose
- Chest X-ray

■ **Table 7.6** Clinical and ECG features suggesting sino-atrial disease or ventricular tachycardia as causes of syncope

Sino-atrial disease

- Clustering of attacks
- Syncope at rest
- Facial pallor during the attack with subsequent flushing
- ECG: may show sinus bradycardia, sinus arrhythmia, sinus pauses, variable P-wave morphology, atrial extrasystoles, episodes of supraventricular tachycardia

Ventricular tachycardia

- Previous myocardial infarction or other ventricular disease
- Syncope during or after exertion
- May complicate anti-arrhythmic therapy (torsade de pointes, p. 15)
- ECG: evidence of infarction; long QT interval

8   Acute confusional state

- Consider in any patient labelled as difficult, uncooperative or a 'poor historian'.
- Usually caused by acute illness (most commonly infection) or an adverse effect of drugs (Appendix 1).

Priorities

1 Assess the mental state: does the patient have an acute confusional state?
- **Check for clouding of consciousness**: reduced alertness, impaired attention and concentration; **disorientation of time** (and often also of place and person); and **impaired short-term memory** (Appendix 2).
- Vivid visual or auditory hallucinations suggest alcohol withdrawal (see below).
- Features distinguishing acute confusional state from dementia and acute functional psychosis are given in Table 8.1.
- Patients with dementia are especially prone to develop confusional states in response to acute illness.

2 Check the drug chart: many drugs may cause an acute confusional state in the elderly, notably benzodiazepines, tricyclics and drugs for parkinsonism.

3 Examine the patient for evidence of acute illness. Specific points to be covered are given in Table 8.2. **Investigations required urgently** are given in Table 8.3.
- Consider non-convulsive status epilepticus if there are mild clonic movements of the eyelids, face or hands, or simple automatism. Diazepam (Diazemuls) (10 mg IV) may terminate the status with improvement in conscious level. Seek expert advice from a neurologist.

■ **Table 8.1** Clinical features of acute confusional state, dementia and acute functional psychosis

Characteristic	Acute confusional state	Dementia	Acute functional psychosis
Onset	Sudden	Insidious	Sudden
Course over 24 hours	Fluctuating, nocturnal exacerbation	Stable	Stable
Consciousness	Reduced	Clear	Clear
Attention	Globally disordered	Normal, except in severe cases	May be disordered
Orientation	Usually impaired	Often impaired	May be impaired
Cognition	Globally impaired	Globally impaired	May be selectively impaired
Hallucinations	Usually visual, or visual and auditory	Often absent	Predominantly auditory
Delusions	Fleeting, poorly systematized	Often absent	Sustained, systematized
Psychomotor activity	Increased, reduced, or shifting unpredictably	Often normal	Varies from psychomotor retardation to severe hyperactivity
Speech	Often incoherent, slow or rapid	Difficulty finding words, perseveration	Normal, slow or rapid
Involuntary movements	Often asterixis or coarse tremor	Often absent	Usually absent
Physical illness or drug toxicity	One or both present	Often absent	Usually absent

Reference:
Lipowski ZJ. Delirium in the elderly patient. *N Engl J Med* 1989; 320: 578–82.
Reproduced by permission of *The New England Journal of Medicine*.

■ **Table 8.2** Examination in acute confusional state

1 Check the pulse, BP and respiratory rate
2 Check for signs of infection:
- Fever or reduced temperature (rectal temperature more reliable in the confused patient if feasible)
- Neck stiffness
- Focal chest signs
- Abdominal tenderness/rigidity
- Cellulitis

3 Are there focal neurological signs? As a minimum, check:
- Pupils ·
- ?Facial asymmetry
- Limb power – ?lateralized weakness
- Tendon reflexes and plantar responses

4 Check for signs suggesting hepatic encephalopathy:
- Stigmata of chronic liver disease
- Asterixis (liver 'flap')

5 In patients with suspected alcohol abuse, check for signs of Wernicke's encephalopathy:
- Nystagmus
- VI nerve palsy (unable to abduct the eye)
- Ataxia (wide-based gait; may be unable to stand or walk)

6 Check for urinary retention and faecal impaction

■ **Table 8.3** Urgent investigation in acute confusional state

- **Blood glucose** (initially by stick test on the ward)
- **Urea, sodium and potassium**
- **Plasma calcium** in patients with malignancy
- **Full blood count**
- **Prothrombin time** if suspected liver disease
- **Blood culture** if temperature is < 36 or $> 37.5°C$ or cannot be measured accurately
- **Urine stick test, microscopy and culture**
- **ECG** if age > 50
- **Chest X-ray** if new focal signs, tachypnoea or fever
- **Arterial blood gases and pH** if cyanosed or chest signs

■ **Table 8.4** Causes of a confusional state associated with alcohol abuse

- Hypoglycaemia (p. 249)
- Acute intoxication
- Alcohol withdrawal (Table 8.5)
- Wernicke's encephalopathy
- Head injury
- Chronic subdural haematoma
- Alcoholic hepatitis
- Hepatic encephalopathy (p. 231)
- Acute pancreatitis
- Alcoholic ketoacidosis (Table 63.3, p. 398)
- Other illness, particularly pneumonia

Further management

1 Specific treatment is directed at the underlying cause.

2 Sedation should only be used if the patient is at risk of self-injury or if aggressive behaviour prevents treatment. Oral administration (syrup may be easier than tablets) is usually preferable to IM or IV. Options include:

- **Haloperidol**, 0.5–10 mg 8–12-hourly PO/IM;
- **thioridazine**, in the elderly start at a dose of 12.5–25 mg at night or 12-hourly PO;
- **chlormethiazole**, PO or by IV infusion (see Table 8.6, p. 71) is specifically indicated for confusional states due to alcohol or drug withdrawal.

Problems

Confusional state associated with alcohol abuse

- Causes to consider are given in Table 8.4. Clinical features of withdrawal are listed in Table 8.5.

■ **Table 8.5** Clinical features that may occur with alcohol withdrawal

Time after stopping drinking	Features
Within 6–12 hours	Tremor, sweating, anorexia, nausea, insomnia, anxiety ('morning shakes') Mild confusional state with agitation
Within 48 hours	'Rum fits': one to six tonic–clonic fits without focal features occurring within a 6-hour period (p. 224)
After 72 hours	Delirium tremens (DT) with tremor, severe confusional state, agitation, visual and auditory hallucinations, and paranoid ideation Tachycardia, sweating and fever

Management of alcohol withdrawal

• **General supportive measures:** fluid replacement if needed; exclusion of hypoglycaemia; treatment of intercurrent illness; vitamin supplements (oral strong compound vitamin B − 2 tablets, plus thiamine 100 mg 12-hourly, and vitamin C − 50 mg 12-hourly).

• **Wernicke's encephalopathy** should be treated with IV thiamine (Parentrovite) one pair of ampoules daily for 5−7 days, given over 10 min; anaphylactic reactions have occurred.

• **Rum fits** are typically self-limiting and do not require specific treatment (p. 224).

• **Drug treatment:** if there is delirium tremens or severe agitation, start chlormethiazole IV (Table 8.6). Otherwise, start either chlormethiazole or chlordiazepoxide PO.

• **Arrange appropriate follow-up** (e.g. referral to an alcohol-problems clinic).

■ **Table 8.6** Chlormethiazole in the management of alcohol withdrawal

Oral regimen using 192 mg capsules* (1 capsule is equivalent to 5 ml of syrup)

Day	Dose
1	3 capsules, 6-hourly
2	2 capsules, 6-hourly
3 and 4	2 capsules, 8-hourly
5 and 6	2 capsules, 12-hourly
7 and 8	2 capsules, at night
Subsequently	Nil

Intravenous regimen (0.8% infusion)

- Start at 60 standard drops per min (4 ml/min)
- When the patient becomes drowsy, reduce to the minimum rate at which mild sedation is maintained (usually 8–15 drops/min)
- Monitor respiratory rate and oxygen saturation by pulse oximetry: stop the infusion if respiratory rate falls below 10/min or Sao_2 is $< 90\%$

* Reduced doses are necessary in patients with hepatic impairment (stigmata or prolonged prothrombin time). Initially give one capsule only and observe the response.

Appendix 1

■ **Table 8.7** Causes of an acute confusional state

Systemic illness

- Infection, usually of the urinary or respiratory tract. Endocarditis and biliary tract sepsis should be considered in the febrile patient without localizing signs
- Organ failure
- Metabolic/endocrine disease

Primary neurological disease

- Postictal state
- Non-dominant parietal lobe stroke
- Subarachnoid haemorrhage (p. 200)

Continued on p. 72

■ **Table 8.7** (Continued)

Primary neurological disease (continued)

- Non-convulsive status epilepticus
- Viral encephalitis (p. 210)

Drugs, notably:

- Benzodiazepines (acute effect and withdrawal)
- Tricyclics
- Drugs for parkinsonism

Alcohol-related (see Tables 8.4 and 8.5, pp. 69, 70)

- Acute intoxication
- Alcohol withdrawal

Urinary retention and faecal impaction

Appendix 2

■ **Table 8.8** Abbreviated mental-status examination of the elderly

1 Age
2 Time (to nearest hour)
3 Address for recall at end of test – this should be repeated by the patient to ensure it has been heard correctly: 42 West Street
4 Year
5 Name of institution
6 Recognition of 2 people (doctor, nurse, etc)
7 Date of birth (day and month sufficient)
8 Year of World War I
9 Name of present Monarch
10 Count backwards 20–1

Each correct answer scores one mark. Healthy elderly people score 8–10

Reference:
Qureshi KN, Hodkinson HM. Evaluation of a ten-question mental test in the institutionalized elderly. *Age and Ageing* 1974; 3: 152–7.

9 Headache

Priorities

On the basis of the clinical assessment (Table 9.1), the patient with headache can be placed in one of five groups:

1 no abnormal signs;
2 local signs;
3 febrile, but no focal neurological signs;
4 papilloedema but no focal neurological signs;
5 reduced conscious level and/or focal neurological signs.

■ **Table 9.1** Clinical assessment of the patient with headache

History

- Is the headache acute, or chronic and recurrent?
- If acute, was the onset sudden?
- Associated loss of consciousness?
- Distribution (unilateral, diffuse, localized)?
- Associated visual symptoms (blurring, transient blindness, scotomata, fortification spectra)?
- Recent travel abroad? (Consider malaria and typhoid, p. 302)
- Is the patient immunocompromised?

Examination

- Temperature
- BP
- Conscious level
- Neck stiffness?
- Focal neurological signs?
- Visual acuity and fields
- Fundi (?papilloedema, ?retinal haemorrhages)
- Sinus tenderness?
- Temporal artery thickening or tenderness?

‎

■ **Table 9.2** Causes of headache with no abnormal signs

- Muscle contraction ('tension') headache
- Migraine
- Drugs (e.g. nitrates, calcium antagonists)
- Toxin exposure (e.g. carbon monoxide poisoning)
- Temporal arteritis
- Subarachnoid haemorrhage (p. 200)
- Thunderclap headache
- Coital cephalgia
- Hyponatraemia (p. 265)

No abnormal signs (Table 9.2)

- **Migraine** is diagnosed on the history of a recurrent throbbing headache with headache-free intervals, and two or more of the following features: **(a)** prodromal visual, sensory or motor symptoms; **(b)** nausea; **(c)** unilateral distribution; **(d)** family history of similar headache. The first migraine headache usually occurs from age 10–30 years. Treatment of acute migraine is given in Table 9.3.
- **Carbon monoxide poisoning** is confirmed by a venous blood carboxyhaemoglobin level > 10%. Management is given on p. 103.
- **Temporal arteritis** should be considered in any patient aged > 50. **Check the erythrocyte sedimentation rate (ESR)** (see above).
- **Subarachnoid haemorrhage** (SAH) should be excluded by cerebrospinal fluid (CSF) examination in patients with **unexplained headache of sudden onset**. Xanthochromia is the most reliable method of differentiating between SAH and traumatic tap, and is always found 12 hours to 2 weeks after SAH. Lumbar puncture should therefore be delayed > 12 hours after the onset of headache unless meningitis is a possibility.
- **Thunderclap headache.** This is a recognized syndrome of sudden severe headache with a benign prognosis, although it may be followed by tension headache or migraine. It can only be reliably distinguished from subarachnoid haemorrhage by normal computed tomography (CT) scan and CSF examination.
- **Coital cephalgia** is a severe headache beginning suddenly during coitus or immediately after orgasm, and is more common in men than

■ **Table 9.3** Treatment of acute migraine

• **Analgesic:** dispersible aspirin or paracetamol
• **Anti-emetic:** metoclopramide 10 mg IM

If the headache does not respond to analgesic, use either:

• **Ergotamine** (contraindicated in patients with vascular disease or hypertension) 2 mg PO; **or**
• **Sumatriptan** (contraindicated in patients with ischaemic heart disease or variant angina) 100 mg PO or 6 mg SC (**not** IV)

women. The prognosis is benign. Subarachnoid haemorrhage must be excluded by CT scan and CSF examination.

• **Hyponatraemia** may cause headache, nausea, vomiting and weakness. Management is given in Chapter 41, p. 265.

Local signs

Acute sinusitis

• Suspect from associated fever, facial pain especially on bending over, mucopurulent nasal discharge and tenderness on pressure over the affected sinus.

• Obtain X-rays of the sinuses (to look for mucosal thickening, a fluid level or opacification).

• Discuss management with an ENT surgeon.

Acute angle-closure glaucoma

• Suspect from blurred vision with reduced visual acuity due to corneal clouding, red eye, pupil fixed in the mid position.

• Refer urgently to an ophthalmologist.

Temporal arteritis

• Consider in any patient over 50 with headache.

• Associated symptoms include malaise, weight loss, jaw claudication, scalp tenderness and visual changes (amaurosis fugax, diplopia and partial or complete loss of vision).

- If the ESR is > 50 mm/hour and/or the temporal artery is thickened or tender (feel 2 cm above and 2 cm forward from the external auditory meatus), start prednisolone. For patients without visual symptoms, give 40 mg daily; with visual symptoms, give 60–80 mg daily.
- Arrange for a temporal-artery biopsy to be done within 48 hours.

Cervical spondylosis
- Suspect from subacute occipital headache associated with pain on rotation of the neck.
- Check for signs of root or cord compression (p. 211).
- X-ray the cervical spine. Treat with an non-steroidal anti-inflammatory drug (NSAID).

Febrile but no focal neurological signs (Table 9.4)

Neck stiffness present
- A lumbar puncture should be performed to exclude **meningitis** (p. 204) or **subarachnoid haemorrhage** (p. 200).

No neck stiffness
- Lumbar puncture is indicated in immunocompromised patients. Neck stiffness is not an invariable feature of **cryptococcal meningitis** (p. 209).
- Consider **encephalitis** (p. 210).
- Consider **malaria** and **typhoid** in patients who have returned from abroad (p. 302).

■ **Table 9.4** Causes of headache with fever but no focal neurological signs

- Meningitis (p. 204)
- Encephalitis (p. 210)
- Acute sinusitis
- Malaria and typhoid (p. 302)
- Other infectious diseases including benign viral illnessess
- Subarachnoid haemorrhage (p. 200)

■ **Table 9.5** Causes of headache with papilloedema but no focal neurological signs

- Accelerated-phase hypertension
- Brain tumour (e.g. in non-dominant frontal lobe)
- Benign intracranial hypertension

Papilloedema but no focal neurological signs (Table 9.5)

- If the diastolic BP is > 120 mmHg and there are retinal haemorrhages or exudates, start antihypertensive therapy (p. 132).
- If the BP is normal, discuss further management with a neurologist.

Reduced conscious level and/or focal neurological signs (Table 9.6)

- The mode of onset of symptoms will help distinguish between vascular (acute onset), infectious (subacute) and neoplastic (chronic) disease.
- If the patient is febrile, take blood cultures and start antibiotic therapy to cover **bacterial meningitis** (p. 204). A CT scan should be performed before lumbar puncture.
- Discuss further management with a neurologist.

■ **Table 9.6** Causes of headache with reduced conscious level and/or focal neurological signs

- Stroke (p. 189)
- Subarachnoid haemorrhage (p. 200)
- Chronic subdural haematoma
- Meningitis (p. 204)
- Encephalitis (p. 210)
- Cerebral malaria (p. 307)
- Brain abscess
- Subdural empyema
- Brain tumour

10 Sepsis and sepsis syndrome

• **Make a working diagnosis of sepsis syndrome** (Table 10.1) if a patient has unexplained **hypotension, oliguria or confusional state** associated with **fever or reduced body temperature ($< 36°C$).**

• *Escherichia coli*, *Staphylococcus aureus* and *epidermidis*, and *Streptococcus pneumoniae* (*pneumococcus*) are the commonest pathogens.

Priorities

1 If systolic BP is $< 90\,mmHg$, give **colloid IV** 500 ml over $15-30\,min$ and **oxygen** 35%. See p. 34 for further management of hypotension.

2 Examine for a possible focus of infection. The clinical setting may make it obvious, e.g. recent instrumentation of urinary or biliary tract. Check for neck stiffness, focal lung crackles or bronchial breathing, heart murmur, abdominal tenderness or guarding, arthritis and soft-tissue abscess. **Obtain a surgical opinion** if you suspect an abdominal or pelvic source of sepsis.

3 Investigations required urgently are given in **Table 10.2**.

4 Start antibiotic therapy as soon as blood has been taken for culture. Guidelines are given in **Table 10.3**. Take into account previous isolates from the patient and the local pattern of antibiotic resistance. In patients with hospital-acquired sepsis:

  • substitute aztreonam or ciprofloxacin for gentamicin if genta-micin resistance is prevalent;

  • substitute vancomycin for flucloxacillin if methicillin-resistant *Staphylococcus aureus* (MRSA) infection is possible. Serum levels of vancomycin should be measured.

5 Transfer the patient to the intensive-therapy unit if:

  • Pao_2 is $< 8\,kPa$ ($60\,mmHg$) despite an inspired oxygen concentration of 35%; or

  • systolic BP is $< 90\,mmHg$ after fluid replacement (i.e. septic shock).

■ **Table 10.1** Diagnosis of sepsis syndrome

Condition	Definition
Sepsis	**Clinical evidence of infection**
Sepsis syndrome	**Sepsis plus altered organ perfusion**
Septic shock	**Sepsis syndrome plus hypotension unresponsive to fluid therapy**

■ **Table 10.2** Urgent investigation of the patient with sepsis and septic shock

- **Full blood count** (the white-cell count may be low in overwhelming bacterial sepsis; low platelet count may reflect disseminated intravascular coagulation, p. 83)
- **Clotting screen** if purpura, prolonged oozing from puncture sites, bleeding from surgical wounds or low platelet count
- **Urea, sodium and potassium**
- **Glucose** (hypoglycaemia can complicate sepsis, especially in patients with liver disease)
- **Amylase** (if abdominal pain/tenderness)
- **Chest X-ray**
- **Arterial gases and pH**
- **Blood culture** (2 sets)*
- **Urine microscopy and culture**
- **Cerebrospinal fluid examination** if suspected meningitis (p. 204)
- **Joint aspiration** if suspected septic arthritis (p. 291)
- **Blood film for malaria** if recent travel to or through an endemic area
- **ECG** if age > 60 or known cardiac disease

* **If suspected IV-line-related sepsis** (central venous line, pulmonary artery catheter, indwelling IV catheter): (a) take blood for culture via the lines and a further sample from a peripheral vein; (b) change the central venous line or pulmonary artery catheter and send the tip for culture.

■ **Table 10.3** 'Blind' antibiotic therapy for sepsis

Suspected primary infection	Antibiotic therapy
Meningitis	Table 30.3, p. 205
Pneumonia	Table 23.4, p. 176
Endocarditis	Gentamicin plus benzylpenicillin
Peritonitis	Cefotaxime plus gentamicin plus metronidazole
Urinary tract	Cefotaxime plus gentamicin
IV-line-related	Gentamicin plus flucloxacillin (see p. 321)
Septic arthritis	Table 47.4, p. 293
Cellulitis	Benzylpenicillin plus flucloxacillin
No localizing signs	
Neutropenic*	Gentamicin plus azlocillin
Other patients	Cefobaxime plus gentamicin plus metronidazole

*See under **Problems** for further management of these patients.
Gentamicin dosages are given in **Appendix 1**.

Problems

Sepsis in the neutropenic patient

- Patients with **neutrophil counts** $< 0.5 \times 10^9$/l are at high risk of bacterial infection, particularly from Gram-negative rods and *Staphylococcus aureus* and *epidermidis*.
- If the neutropenic patient has **a single temperature** $> 38.5°C$, **or three elevations to** $> 38.0°C$ **during a 24-hour period**, the likely cause is bacterial infection and **antibiotic therapy should be started**.
- **Examine for a possible focus of infection.** Examination should include the entire skin, including the perineum and perianal region, indwelling IV line and other IV sites, and the mouth, teeth and sinuses.
- **Investigation** as in **Table 10.2**.

Table 10.4 Common modifications or additions to initial empirical antibiotic therapy in patients with neutropenia and fever

Status or symptoms	Modifications of primary regimen
Fever	
● Persists > 1 week	Add empirical antifungal therapy with amphotericin B
● Recurs after 1 week or later, persistent neutropenia	Add empirical antifungal therapy
● Persists or recurs at time of recovery from neutropenia	Imaging for hepatosplenic candidiasis and evaluate need for antifungal therapy
Blood cultures	
Before antibiotic therapy	
● Gram-positive organism	Add vancomycin pending further identification
● Gram-negative organism	Maintain regimen if patient is stable and isolate is sensitive. If *Pseudomonas aeruginosa*, enterobacter or citrobacter is isolated, add an aminoglycoside or an additional beta-lactam antibiotic
During antibiotic therapy	
● Gram-positive organism	Add vancomycin pending further identification
● Gram-negative organism	Change to new combination regimen (e.g. imipenem + gentamicin or vancomycin, or gentamicin + piperacillin)
Head, eyes, ears, nose and throat	
● Necrotizing or marginal gingivitis	Add anti-anaerobic agent (clindamycin or metronidazole)
● Vesicular or ulcerative lesions	Suspect herpes simplex; culture and begin acyclovir
● Sinus tenderness or nasal ulcerative lesions	Suspect fungal infection with aspergillus or mucor
Gastrointestinal tract	
● Retrosternal burning pain	Suspect *Candida*, herpes simplex or both. Add antifungal and if no response, acyclovir. Bacterial oesophagitis is also a possibility. Consider endoscopy if no response within 48 hours

Continued on p. 82

■ **Table 10.4** *(Continued)*

Status or symptoms	Modifications of primary regimen
• Acute abdominal pain	Suspect typhlitis as well as appendicitis if pain in right lower quadrant. Add anti-anaerobic agent. Obtain surgical opinion
• Perianal tenderness	Add anti-anaerobic agent. Obtain surgical opinion

Respiratory tract

• New focal lesion, recovering from neutropenia	Observe carefully, as this may be a consequence of inflammatory response in concert with neutrophil recovery
• New focal lesion, continuing neutropenia	Aspergillus is the chief concern. Perform appropriate cultures and consider biopsy. If not a candidate for biopsy, give high-dose amphotericin B
• New interstitial pneumonitis	Attempt diagnosis by examination of induced sputum or bronchoalveolar lavage. If not feasible, begin empirical treatment with cotrimoxazole or pentamidine. Consider non-infectious causes and the need for open-lung biopsy if no improvement after 4 days of therapy

Central venous catheters

• Positive culture for organism other than bacillus species or Candida	Attempt to treat. Rotate antibiotic administration in patients with multiple-lumen catheters
• Positive culture for Bacillus species or Candida	Remove catheter and treat appropriately
• Exit-site infection mycobacterium or Aspergillus	Remove catheter and treat appropriately
• Tunnel infection	Remove catheter and treat appropriately

From Pizzo PA. Management of fever in patients with cancer and treatment-induced neutropenia. *N Engl J Med* 1993; 328: 1323–7. Reproduced by permission of *The New England Journal of Medicine*.

● Several **antibiotic regimens** have been shown to be effective in neutropenic patients without localizing signs: an aminoglycoside plus an antipseudomonal penicillin (e.g. gentamicin and azlocillin) or monotherapy with a third generation cephalosporin (e.g. ceftazidime).

● Further management is given in Table 10.4. Obtain expert advice from a haematologist and microbiologist.

Sepsis in the IV drug abuser

● Several causes of fever must be considered (Table 10.5).

● Right-sided endocarditis may not give rise to abnormal cardiac signs.

● If septicaemic, antibiotic therapy must cover staphylococci (see Table 10.3, p. 80).

Sepsis in the patient with HIV/AIDS

See p. 284.

Disseminated intravascular coagulation

● Suspect in patients with purpura, prolonged oozing from puncture sites, or bleeding from surgical wounds.

■ **Table 10.5** Possible causes of fever in the IV drug abuser

● Infection at injection sites
● Thrombophlebitis
● Endocarditis (especially right-sided)
● Pulmonary tuberculosis
● Hepatitis B
● Septic arthritis
● Pyrogen reaction
● AIDS-related infection, e.g. cryptococcal meningitis, pneumocystis carinii pneumonia

- Confirm by a low platelet count, prolonged prothrombin and activated partial thromboplastin times, and increased concentration of fibrin degradation products.
- If there is active bleeding, give fresh frozen plasma and platelets: seek advice from a haematologist.
- Heparin is not of proven benefit.

Appendix 1: gentamicin

- **Aminoglycoside principally active against Gram-negative rods.**
- Can be given IM or IV (the preferred route in severe infection).
- **Loading dose:** based on body weight – give 2 mg/kg.
- **Maintenance dose and dosage interval:** based on renal function. Table 10.6 serves as a guide, but **serum levels should be checked in all patients**.

Serum levels

Trough level reflects the renal excretion of the preceding dose. Take blood just before the next dose. The level should be 1–2 mg/l: if >2 mg/l, decrease the dose or increase the interval between doses.

■ **Table 10.6** Gentamicin dosage

Blood urea (mmol/l)	Dose (mg)		Interval between doses (hours)
	Wt. < 60 kg	> 60 kg	
<7	60	80	8
7–10	60	80	12
11–15	60	80	18
16–20	60	80	24
>20	Check serum level 24 hours after loading dose		

Peak level: reflects the adequacy of the dose. Take blood 1 hour after IM dose or 15–20 min after IV dose. The level should be in the range 5–10 mg/l: increase or decrease the dose as required.

• **Toxic effects (ototoxicity and renal failure)** may occur if trough levels are persistently > 2 or peak levels > 12 mg/l.

11 Poisoning

If you need advice about the management of poisoning, contact a poisons centre (Appendix 1).

Priorities

The unconscious patient

1 Priority management of the unconscious patient is described in detail on p. 53. The key elements are listed below.

- **Establish a clear airway.**
- **Give oxygen** (10 l/min by a tightly fitting facemask if carbon-monoxide poisoning is suspected (Appendix 5)).
- **Endotracheal intubation and ventilation if appropriate** (Table 6.1, p. 54).
- Put in an IV cannula. **Check for and treat hypoglycaemia** (p. 249). Give **naloxone** (Table 6.2, p. 54) if opiate poisoning is suspected.
- Attach an ECG monitor and **correct arrhythmias**.
- Check the BP and **correct hypotension** (p. 34).
- **Control fits** (p. 218).

2 Obtain the history from all available sources: ambulance personnel, relatives, GP and hospital records.

3 Perform a **systematic examination**.

- Points to cover in the neurological examination of the unconscious patient are given in Table 6.4, p. 56.
- The clinical features may give clues to the poison (Table 11.1).
- Is there evidence of substance abuse? Check for needle marks in the antecubital fossae, neck, supraclavicular areas, groins, dorsum of feet and under the tongue.
- Check for complications of coma (hypothermia, pressure area necrosis, corneal abrasions, inhalation pneumonia).

4 Investigation is given in Table 11.2. The results may provide further clues to the toxin.

■ **Table 11.1** Clues to the poison

Feature	Poisons to consider
Coma	Barbiturates, benzodiazepines, ethanol, glutethimide, opiates, trichloroethanol, tricyclics
Fits	Amphetamines, cocaine, dextropropoxyphene, insulin, oral hypoglycaemics, phenothiazines, theophylline, tricyclics
Constricted pupils	Opiates, organophosphates, trichloroethanol
Dilated pupils	Amphetamines, cocaine, glutethimide, phenothiazines, quinine, sympathomimetics, tricyclics
Arrhythmias	Anti-arrhythmics, anticholinergics, phenothiazines, quinine, sympathomimetics, tricyclics
Hypertension	Amphetamines, cocaine
Pulmonary oedema	Carbon monoxide, ethylene glycol, irritant gases, opiates, organophosphates, paraquat, salicylates, tricyclics
Ketones on breath	Ethanol, isopropyl alcohol
Hypothermia	Barbiturates, phenothiazines, tricyclics
Hyperthermia	Amphetamines, anticholinergics, cocaine, MAO inhibitors
Hypoglycaemia	Insulin, oral hypoglycaemics, ethanol, salicylates
Hyperglycaemia	Theophylline, organophosphates, salbutamol
Renal failure (not due to hypotension or rhabdomyolysis)	Amanita phalloides, ethylene glycol, paracetamol, salicylates
Hypokalaemia	Salbutamol, salicylates, theophylline
Metabolic acidosis	Carbon monoxide, ethanol, ethylene glycol, methanol, paracetamol, salicylates, tricyclics
Raised plasma osmolality	Ethanol, ethylene glycol, isopropyl alcohol, methanol

MAO, Monoamine oxidase.

■ **Table 11.2** Urgent investigation of the unconscious patient with suspected poisoning

- Blood glucose
- Urea, sodium and potassium
- Plasma osmolality*
- Paracetamol and salicylate levels (as mixed poisoning is common)
- Full blood count
- Arterial blood gases and pH
- Chest X-ray
- ECG if there is hypotension, coexistent heart disease, suspected ingestion of cardiotoxic drugs (anti-arrhythmics, tricyclics) or age > 60

- **If the substance ingested is not known, save serum** (10 ml), **urine** (50 ml) **and vomitus or first gastric aspirate** (50 ml) at 4°C in case later analysis is needed

* The normal range of plasma osmolality is 280–300 mosmol/kg.
If the measured plasma osmolality (by freezing-point-depression method) exceeds calculated osmolality (from the formula [2(Na + K) + urea + glucose]) by 10 mosmol/kg or more, consider poisoning with ethanol, ethylene glycol, isopropyl alcohol or methanol.

The conscious patient

1 Check baseline observations: conscious level (fully orientated or confused), pulse, BP, respiratory rate, temperature, and blood glucose by stick test if indicated.

2 Establish:
- which poisons were taken, in what amount, and over what period;
- whether the patient has vomited since ingestion;
- the symptoms;
- associated physical or psychiatric illness.

3 Investigations required will depend on the poisons and the presence of other physical illness. After poisoning with some drugs (Table 11.3) **plasma levels** should be checked.

■ **Table 11.3** Poisoning in which plasma levels should be measured

Poison	Plasma level at which specific treatment is indicated	Treatment
Aspirin and other salicylates	Appendix 3	
Barbiturates	Discuss with Poisons Centre	
Digoxin	> 4 ng/ml (> 5 nmol/l)	p. 27
Ethylene glycol	> 500 mg/l	HD, PD
Iron	> 3.5 mg/l*	Desferrioxamine
Lithium (plain tube)	> 5 mmol/l	HD, PD
Methanol	> 500 mg/l	HD, PD
Paracetamol	Appendix 4	
Theophylline	> 50 mg/l	RAC, HP

HD, Haemodialysis; HP, haemoperfusion; PD, peritoneal dialysis; RAC, repeated activated charcoal.
* Also measure level if clinical evidence of severe toxicity (hypotension, nausea, vomiting, diarrhoea) or if massive ingestion (> 200 mg elemental iron/kg body weight; one 200 mg tablet of ferrous sulphate contains 60 mg elemental iron).
NB: Always check the **units of measurement** used by the laboratory.

Further management

Reducing absorption

1 Activated charcoal (50 g mixed with 200 ml of water) should be given if a significant amount of any drug or poison has been ingested within 2 hours and gastric lavage or oral antidotes (Appendix 2) are not indicated. Exceptions to this are poisoning with alcohols, glycols, iron or lithium (which do not bind to activated charcoal).
2 Gastric lavage should be performed if a potentially dangerous dose has been ingested within 4 hours (or within 8 hours in the case of salicylates or if the drug delays gastric emptying) (Table 11.4), or the patient is unconscious and the time of ingestion is not known.

■ **Table 11.4** Indications for gastric lavage

Drug or poison	Amount ingested (in adults)	Time within which lavage must be performed (hours)
Aspirin	> 10 g	12
Benzodiazepines	Lavage not indicated*	
Cyanide	Any case with symptoms	1
Dextropropoxyphene	> 325 mg	4
Digoxin	> 5 mg	4
Ethylene glycol	> 100 ml	4
Methanol	> 25 ml	4
Paracetamol	> 7.5 g (5 g†)	4
Phenobarbitone	> 1000 mg	8
Phenytoin	Lavage not indicated*	
Theophylline	> 2.5 g	4 (8‡)
Tricyclics	> 750 mg	8
Valproate	Lavage not indicated*	

* Except in massive overdose, when each case should be considered on its merits.
† If hepatic enzyme induction is likely from chronic alcohol abuse or drug therapy (carbamazepine, phenobarbitone, phenytoin, rifampicin).
‡ If sustained release preparation taken.

• **Gastric lavage should not be performed: (a)** after ingestion of corrosives (acids, alkalis, kettle descaler, bleach); **(b)** after ingestion of petroleum derivatives (petrol, paraffin, 'turps substitute', white spirit and kerosene), unless the airway is protected by a cuffed endotracheal tube to prevent aspiration pneumonitis; or **(c)** in patients with oesophageal varices or stricture, or previous gastric surgery.

• The procedure is described in Table 11.5: if the patient is conscious, verbal consent must be obtained. If unconscious, a cuffed endotracheal tube should be inserted first (by an anaesthetist) to protect the airway.

3 Induced emesis with ipecacuanha is not of benefit in adults and **should not be used.**

■ **Table 11.5** Technique of gastric lavage

- If the patient is unconscious, a cuffed endotracheal tube should be inserted first to protect the airway
- Suction apparatus should be to hand
- Tip the trolley head down, with the patient lying on his or her left side
- Use a wide-bore tube (Jacques gauge 30 in adults) that has been lubricated (e.g. with KY jelly)
- Insert the tube. The gastro-oesophageal junction is about 40 cm from the incisor teeth. Confirm that it is in the stomach by aspirating and test with litmus paper
- Run in 300–600 ml of water warmed to body temperature and then drain out. Repeat 3–4 times or more if the washings still contain tablets
- Leave activated charcoal (50 g in 200 ml water) in the stomach, unless contraindicated (poisoning with alcohols, glycols, iron or lithium)

■ **Table 11.6** Drugs whose elimination is increased by repeated dosing with activated charcoal

- Amitriptyline
- Aspirin and other salicylates
- Carbamazepine
- Dapsone
- Digoxin and digitoxin
- Phenobarbitone and other barbiturates
- Phenytoin
- Quinine
- Sustained-release preparations
- Theophylline
- Tricyclics

Increasing elimination

1 Drugs whose elimination can be increased by **repeated dosing with activated charcoal** are given in Table 11.6.

- Give 50 g initially then 25 g 4-hourly PO or nasogastric tube until recovery or until plasma drug levels have fallen to within the safe range.

2 Other methods may be indicated in selected cases (see Table 11.3,

p. 89). Discuss management with a poisons centre. **Is a specific antidote or treatment indicated?**

• See **Appendix 2. Discuss the case with a poisons centre** first,
unless you are familiar with the poison and its antidote, as some
antidotes may be harmful if given inappropriately.

• The management of **aspirin, paracetamol and carbon monoxide
poisoning** is given in **Appendices 3, 4 and 5**.

Supportive treatment

1 Monitoring of the patient with severe poisoning is given in Table
11.7.

• If the patient has an endotracheal tube, transfer to the intensive-
therapy unit. Place a nasogastric tube to prevent gastric dilatation.

• Unconscious patients not requiring intubation should be nursed
in the lateral semiprone position in a high-dependency area.

2 Management of problems commonly seen with poisoning is outlined in Table 11.8.

■ **Table 11.7** Monitoring of the patient with severe poisoning

In all patients (initial frequency of observation)

• Conscious level (hourly)
• Respiratory rate (every 15 min)
• Oxygen saturation by pulse oximeter (continuous display)
• ECG monitor (continuous display)
• BP (every 15 min)
• Temperature (hourly)

In selected patients

• **Urine output via catheter** if poison potentially nephrotoxic, forced diuresis
indicated, patient hypotensive or comatose
• **Arterial blood gases and pH** if poison can cause metabolic acidosis (see
Table 11.2, p. 88) or there is suspected acute respiratory distress syndrome
(p. 140) or after inhalation injury
• **Blood glucose** if poison may cause hypo- or hyperglycaemia (see Table 11.1,
p. 87) or in paracetamol poisoning presenting after 16 hours

■ Table 11.8 Problems encountered in the patient with poisoning

Problem	Comment and management
Hypotension	Usually reflects vasodilatation, but always consider other causes (e.g. gastrointestinal bleeding). Obtain an ECG if the patient is aged > 60, has known cardiac disease or has taken a cardiotoxic poison. See p. 34 for further management
Arrhythmias	Due to toxin or metabolic complications: check arterial gases and pH, and plasma potassium. See p. 9 for further management
Respiratory depression	Half-life of most opiates is longer than that of naloxone and repeated doses or an infusion may be required (Table 6.2, p. 54). Elective ventilation may be preferable
Inhalation pneumonia	Treatment includes tracheobronchial suction, physiotherapy and antibiotic therapy (Table 23.4, p. 176)
Coma	If associated with focal signs, intracranial haematoma must be excluded by computed tomography
Cerebral oedema	May occur after cardiac arrest or severe carbon monoxide poisoning, or in fulminant hepatic failure due to paracetamol (p. 231). Results in hypertension and dilated pupils. Give mannitol 20% 100−200 ml (0.5 g/kg) IV over 10 min, provided urine output is >30 ml/hour. Check plasma osmolality: further mannitol may be given until plasma osmolality is 320 mosmol/kg. Hyperventilate to an arterial P_{CO_2} of 4 kPa (30 mmHg)
Fits	Due to toxin or metabolic complications. Check blood glucose, arterial gases and pH, plasma sodium and potassium. See p. 218 for drug therapy and further management
Renal failure	May be due to prolonged hypotension, nephrotoxic poison, haemolysis or rhabdomyolysis. See p. 238 for further management
Gastric stasis	Nasogastric tube should be placed in comatose patients to reduce the risk of regurgitation and inhalation
Hypothermia	Manage by passive rewarming (Table 45.4, p. 281)

Psychiatric assessment

- This should be performed when the patient has recovered from the physical effects of the poisoning.
- Points to be covered are given in Table 11.9.
- Patients at increased risk of suicide (Table 11.10) and those with overt psychiatric illness should be discussed with a psychiatrist.
- Follow-up by the GP or psychiatric services should be arranged before discharge.

■ **Table 11.9** Psychiatric assessment after self-poisoning

- **Circumstances of the overdose:** carefully planned, indecisive or impulsive? Taken alone or in the presence of another person? Action taken to avoid intervention or discovery? Suicidal intent admitted?

- **Past history** of self-poisoning or self-injury? Psychiatric history or contact with psychiatric services? Alcohol or substance abuse?

- **Family history** of depression or suicide?

- **Social circumstances?**

- **Mental state:** evidence of depression or psychosis?

■ **Table 11.10** Patients at high risk of suicide after self-poisoning

- Middle-aged or elderly male
- Widowed/divorced/separated
- Unemployed
- Living alone
- Chronic physical illness
- Psychiatric illness, especially depression
- Alcohol or substance abuse
- Circumstances of poisoning: massive; planned; taken alone; timed so that intervention or discovery unlikely; suicidal intent admitted

Appendix 1: poisons centres

■ Table 11.11 Poisons centres

City	Telephone
Belfast	01232 240503
Birmingham	0121 5543801
Cardiff	01222 709901
Dublin	010 3531 379964 or 010 3531 379966
Edinburgh	0131 2292477 or 0131 2282441
Leeds	0113 2430715 or 0113 2432799
London	0171 6359191
Newcastle	0191 2325131

Appendix 2: specific antidotes

■ Table 11.12 Specific antidotes

Poison	Antidote
Anticholinergic agents	**Physostigmine** 1–2 mg IV over 5 min. Use only for severe delirium. May be useful to treat fits or tachyarrhythmias
Arsenic	**Dimercaprol** 2.5–5 mg/kg by deep IM injection 4-hourly for 2 days then 2.5 mg/kg 12-hourly on day 3 then 2.5 mg/kg once daily
Benzodiazepines	**Flumazenil** 0.2 mg IV over 30 s. If there is no response after 30 s, give 0.3 mg over 30 s. If there is no response after 30 s, give 0.5 mg over 30 s at 1-min intervals up to a total dose of 3 mg. Should not be given if the patient has also taken tricyclics or was taking benzodiazepines for epilepsy
Beta-blockers	**Glucagon** 5–10 mg IV. Titrate to response. Maintenance dose of 2–10 mg/hour by IV infusion may be used
Calcium antagonists	**Calcium gluconate** 10 ml of 10% solution slowly IV. Monitor ECG. Repeat if needed. Check calcium after third dose

Continued on p. 96

■ **Table 11.12** *(Continued)*

Poison	Antidote
Cyanide	**Dicobalt edetate** 600 mg IV over 1 min then 300 mg if recovery does not occur within 1 min, or **sodium nitrite** 10 ml of 3% solution IV over 3 min followed by **sodium thiosulphate** 25 ml of 50% solution IV over 10 min
Digoxin	**Digoxin-specific antibody fragments** (Table 2.14, p. 28)
Ethylene glycol	**Ethanol.** Loading dose 10 ml/kg of 10% solution in normal saline IV, followed by 0.15 ml/kg/hour. Double maintenance dose should be used during dialysis. Titrate to a plasma ethanol level of 1 g/l (22 mmol/l)
Fluoride	**Calcium gluconate** 10−20 g in 25 ml water PO then 10 ml of 10% solution slowly IV
Iron	**Desferrioxamine** 5 mg/kg by slow IV injection
Lead	**Dimercaprol** (see under arsenic) or **Penicillamine** 250 mg − 2 g PO daily
Mercury	**Dimercaprol** (see under arsenic) or **Penicillamine** (see under lead)
Methanol	**Ethanol** (see under ethylene glycol)
Opiates	**Naloxone** (see Table 6.2, p. 54)
Organophosphates	**Atropine** 1.2−2.4 mg IV every 10 min until heart rate >75/min and mouth dry. Give further doses for 2−3 days
Paracetamol	**Acetylcysteine** or **Methionine** (Appendix 4)
Paraquat	**Fuller's Earth** 250 ml of 30% suspension PO 4-hourly for 24−48 hours. Give with magnesium sulphate as a purgative (250 ml of 5% solution until diarrhoea occurs)
Thallium	**Prussian blue** 10 g 12-hourly PO with a magnesium sulphate purgative (see under paraquat) until thallium is no longer detected in the faeces
Warfarin	**Vitamin K** or **fresh frozen plasma** (see Table 60.14, p. 389)

NB: Discuss the case with a poisons information centre first, unless you are familiar with the poison and its antidote, as some antidotes may be harmful if given inappropriately.

Appendix 3: poisoning with aspirin and other salicylates

• Ingestion of $> 10\,g$ of aspirin may cause moderate or severe poisoning in an adult.
• Clinical features of severe poisoning include tremor, tinnitus, hyperventilation, nausea, vomiting, and sweating.

Priorities

1 Gastric lavage should be performed if the patient is seen within 12 hours of ingestion of $> 10\,g$, followed by repeated dosing with activated charcoal.
2 Investigation is given in Table 11.13. Further management depends on the plasma salicylate level (Table 11.14).

Further management

Mild poisoning
• Fluid replacement (PO or IV).

Moderate or severe poisoning
• Fluid replacement, preferably guided by measurement of central venous pressure (CVP) if the patient is aged over 60 or has cardiac disease.
• Urinary catheter to monitor urine output.
• Correct hypokalaemia with IV potassium.
• Correct hypoglycaemia with IV dextrose.
• Give vitamin K 10 mg IV to reverse hypoprothrombinaemia.
• Patients with moderate poisoning should be managed with urinary alkalinization **(Fig. 11.1)**.
• Patients with severe or massive poisoning (plasma level $> 750\,mg/l$ ($> 5.4\,mmol/l$) after rehydration or $> 1000\,mg/l$ ($>7.2\,mmol/l$) before rehydration) or renal failure or pulmonary oedema should be referred for haemodialysis. Peritoneal dialysis can be used but is less effective.

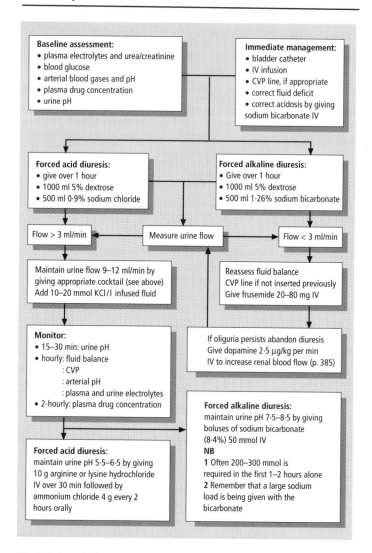

Fig. 11.1 Forced diuresis in adults. From Vale A, Meredith T, Buckley B, *BMJ* 1984; 289: 367.

■ **Table 11.13** Investigation in poisoning with aspirin and other salicylates

- Full blood count
- Prothrombin time (may be prolonged)
- Urea, sodium and potassium (hypokalaemia is common)
- Blood glucose (hypoglycaemia may occur)
- Arterial blood gases and pH (respiratory alkalosis in early stage, progressing to metabolic acidosis)
- Plasma salicylate level (sample taken >6 hours after ingestion) (see Table 11.14)
- Chest X-ray (pulmonary oedema may occur)

■ **Table 11.14** Plasma salicylate level (sample taken >6 hours after ingestion): interpretation and management

Plasma level			
(mg/l)	(mmol/l)	Interpretation	**Action**
150–250	1.1–1.8	Therapeutic	None required
250–500	1.8–3.6	Mild poisoning	Fluid replacement
500–750	3.6–5.4	Moderate poisoning	Urinary alkalinization
750–1000	5.4–7.2	Severe poisoning	Haemodialysis or peritoneal dialysis
>1000	>7.2	Massive poisoning	Haemodialysis or peritoneal dialysis

Appendix 4: paracetamol poisoning

- Ingestion of >7.5 g of paracetamol (>5 g if there is hepatic enzyme induction due to chronic alcohol abuse or drug therapy (carbamazepine, phenobarbitone, phenytoin, rifampicin)) may cause moderate or severe poisoning in an adult.
- Clinical features of severe poisoning: early (<24 hours) none or

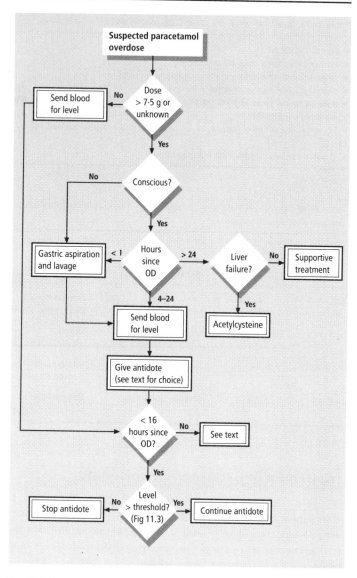

Fig. 11.2 Management of paracetamol poisoning.

nausea and vomiting; late (> 24 hours) nausea and vomiting, right-upper-quadrant pain, jaundice and encephalopathy.

Priorities (Fig. 11.2)

1 Gastric lavage should be performed if the patient is seen within 1 hour of ingestion of > 7.5 g (or > 5 g if hepatic enzyme induction is likely).

2 Send blood for plasma paracetamol level determination at 4 hours after ingestion.

3 Patients who might have taken > 7.5 g (or > 5 g if hepatic enzyme induction is likely) within 24 hours should be treated immediately with oral methionine (if within 12 hours) or IV acetylcysteine (Table 11.15). This can be stopped if the plasma level is below the treatment line **(Fig. 11.3)**, except in patients who present > 16 hours, when the plasma level is not a reliable guide to the need for treatment.

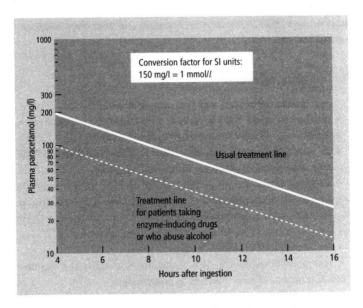

Fig. 11.3 Treatment thresholds in paracetamol poisoning. From Ferner R. *Prescribers' Journal* 1993; 33: 45–50.

■ **Table 11.15** Treatment regimens in paracetamol poisoning

Drug	Regimen
Methionine or **Acetylcysteine**	Supplied as 250 mg tablets
	Give 2.5 g followed by 3 doses of 2.5 g 4-hourly PO
	Supplied as 10 ml ampoules containing 2 gram (200 mg/ml)
	Give 150 mg/kg in 200 ml dextrose 5% over 15 minutes, then
	50 mg/kg in 500 ml 5% dextrose over 4 hours, then
	100 mg/kg in 1 l 5% dextrose over 16 hours by IV infusion

Acetylcysteine should be given: (a) if the overdose is very large or plasma level very high; (b) if activated charcoal has been given; (c) if the patient is vomiting before or after administration of methionine; (d) if the patient is comatose; (e) if the patient is seen > 12 hours after ingestion.

4 Acetylcysteine has also been shown to be of benefit in patients who present more than 24 hours after ingestion and who have fulminant hepatic failure.

Further management

1 Check prothrombin time and plasma creatinine:
- once at 24 hours after ingestion, or after antidote treatment is complete in patients who presented within 8 hours;
- at 24 and 48 hours in patients who presented after 8 hours; if the results are normal, no medical follow-up is needed.

2 Acute liver failure and renal failure (due to acute tubular necrosis) are potential complications of paracetamol poisoning, occurring at 36–72 hours after ingestion. Indications for referral to a liver unit are given in Table 11.16. In such patients (before transfer):
- monitor conscious level 8-hourly;
- start an IV infusion of 5–10% dextrose 1 l 12-hourly and monitor blood glucose 4-hourly – correct hypoglycaemia
- monitor CVP and urine output – correct hypovolaemia with colloid;
- check prothrombin time 12-hourly and plasma creatinine daily;

■ **Table 11.16** Paracetamol poisoning: indications for referral to a liver unit

- Rapid development of grade-2 encephalopathy (confused but able to answer questions)
- Prothrombin time > 45 s at 48 hours or > 50 s at 72 hours
- Increasing plasma creatinine
- Arterial pH < 7.3 more than 24 hours after ingestion

- start prophylaxis against gastric stress ulceration with sucralfate 1 g 6-hourly by mouth or nasogastric tube;
- see Chapter 35 for further management of liver failure.

Appendix 5: carbon monoxide poisoning

- May occur from inhalation of car exhaust fumes, fumes from inadequately maintained or ventilated heating systems (including those using natural gas), smoke from all types of fires, and methylene chloride in paint strippers (by hepatic metabolism).
- The severity of poisoning depends on the concentration of carbon monoxide in the inspired air, the length of exposure and the presence of anaemia or cardiorespiratory disease.
- Clinical features of acute poisoning are given in Table 11.17.

■ **Table 11.17** Acute carbon monoxide poisoning: clinical features

Blood carboxy-haemoglobin (%)	Clinical features which may be seen
< 10	No symptoms – acute poisoning excluded if exposure was within 4 hours
10–50	Headache, nausea, vomiting, tachycardia, tachypnoea
> 50	Coma, fits, cardiorespiratory arrest

Priorities

1 If carbon monoxide poisoning is suspected, give 100% oxygen (10 l/min) using a tightly fitting facemask with a circuit which minimizes rebreathing.

- Unconscious patients should be intubated and ventilated mechanically with 100% oxygen. Cerebral oedema may occur and is treated with mannitol and mild hyperventilation (see Table 11.8, p. 93).

2 Attach an ECG monitor and record a 12-lead ECG. Severe poisoning may result in myocardial ischaemia, with anginal chest pain, ST segment depression and arrhythmias.

3 Check the carboxyhaemoglobin (COHb) level in venous blood (heparinized sample). If acute carbon monoxide poisoning is confirmed (COHb > 10%), recheck hourly and continue 100% oxygen until two consecutive samples contain < 5%.

4 Check arterial blood gases and pH (metabolic acidosis is usually present) and arrange a chest X-ray.

5 If **hyperbaric oxygen therapy** is indicated (Table 11.18), the location of the nearest compression chamber can be obtained from the advisory service run by the Institute of Naval Medicine (telephone 0831 151523).

■ **Table 11.18** Carbon monoxide poisoning: indications for hyperbaric oxygen therapy

- Carboxyhaemoglobin level > 40% at any time
- Coma
- Neurological symptoms or signs other than mild headache
- Evidence of myocardial ischaemia
- Pregnancy

Section 2
Specific Problems

12 Acute myocardial infarction

- **Acute central chest pain (> 30 min duration)** is the commonest symptom but may be absent or overshadowed by other clinical features (Table 12.1), particularly in elderly patients.
- **The working diagnosis is based on the history and ECG (Fig. 12.1).** Confirmation of myocardial infarction requires a two-fold or greater rise in cardiac enzymes (Appendix 1). For prolonged angina without ECG changes of infarction see Chapter 13.
- **Remember that chest or upper abdominal pain with ECG abnormalities can occur in several conditions other than myocardial infarction** (unstable angina, aortic dissection, pericarditis, pulmonary embolism, duodenal perforation, pancreatitis and biliary tract disease).

Priorities

1 Attach an **ECG monitor. Make sure a defibrillator is near because ventricular fibrillation (VF) is a common early complication.**
2 **Give oxygen and put in a peripheral IV cannula.**
3 **Relieve pain with diamorphine.** Give 5 mg (2.5 mg if the patient is small or elderly) IV over 3–5 min, with further doses of 2.5 mg every 10–15 min until pain free. An anti-emetic should also be given (e.g. prochlorperazine 12.5 mg or metoclopramide 10 mg IV).
4 **Record an ECG. Other investigations are given in Table 12.2.**
5 **Give aspirin 300 mg (chewed),** unless the patient is already taking this or it is contraindicated, and nitrate sublingually (1 tablet or 2 puffs of spray).
6 **Is the patient suitable for IV thrombolytic therapy (Tables 12.3–12.6)? If so, this should be given without delay.**
7 **Are there complications of infarction** — pulmonary oedema, hypotension, mitral regurgitation, ventricular septal rupture, arrhythmia or heart block? See **Haemodynamic problems** below.

■ **Table 12.1** Presentations of myocardial infarction without chest pain

- Acute pulmonary oedema
- Syncope (from an arrhythmia)
- Acute epigastric pain and vomiting
- Postoperative hypotension or oliguria
- Acute confusional state
- Stroke
- Diabetic hyperglycaemic states

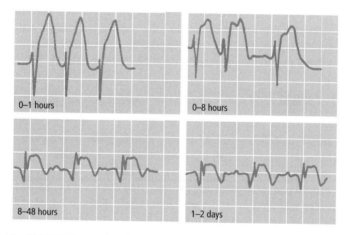

Fig. 12.1 ECG changes in acute myocardial infarction.

Further management

1 Bed rest with ECG monitoring for 24 hours followed by a programme of mobilization.

2 Oxygen can be discontinued if the chest X-ray shows clear lungs and there are no complications of infarction.

3 Prophylaxis against venous and arterial thrombo-embolism.

■ **Table 12.2** Urgent investigation in suspected myocardial infarction

- **ECG** (repeat daily for 3 days or if pain recurs)
- **Chest X-ray** (not essential in patients with definite and uncomplicated myocardial infarction)
- **Urea, sodium and potassium** (recheck potassium if significant arrhythmia occurs or after large diuresis)
- **Blood glucose** by stick test: insulin-dependent diabetes should be managed by insulin infusion (p. 262)

For later analysis

- **Cardiac enzymes** (check daily for 3 days or if pain recurs)
- **Full blood count**
- **Cholesterol** (value is representative if checked within 24 hours of infarction and enables patients with severe hypercholesterolaemia to be identified before discharge)

■ **Table 12.3** Thrombolytic therapy: criteria to be met

- **Clinically definite myocardial infarction**
- **Within 12 hours of the onset of pain** (within 24 hours if chest pain and/or ST elevation are still present and the infarct is large)
- **Regional ST elevation** (>2 mm in chest leads, >1 mm in limb leads); **regional ST depression due to posterior infarction; or left bundle branch block**
- **No contraindication to thrombolysis** (see Table 12.4)

- Patients who are not receiving heparin by infusion should receive heparin 5000 U 8-hourly SC until fully mobile.
- In patients with large Q-wave anterior infarctions, consider warfarin therapy for 3 months as prophylaxis against systemic embolism from left ventricular mural thrombus (see Table 60.13, p. 388 for starting warfarin).

4 On your daily round: (a) ask the patient about further chest pain (Table 12.7); (b) check the temperature chart (Table 12.8); (c) listen to the heart and lungs (Table 12.9).

■ **Table 12.4** Thrombolytic therapy: contraindications

Absolute

- Active internal bleeding
- Suspected aortic dissection
- Prolonged or traumatic cardiopulmonary resuscitation
- Recent head trauma or known intracranial neoplasm
- Trauma or surgery within the previous 2 weeks which could be a source of rebleeding
- Diabetic haemorrhagic retinopathy or other haemorrhagic ophthalmic condition
- Pregnancy
- Previous allergic reaction to streptokinase or anistreplase (in which case use alteplase)
- Recorded BP > 200/120 mmHg
- History of cerebrovascular accident known to be haemorrhagic

Relative

- Recent trauma or surgery (> 2 weeks)
- History of chronic severe hypertension with or without drug therapy
- Active peptic ulcer
- History of cerebrovascular accident
- Known bleeding diathesis or current use of anticoagulants
- Significant liver dysfunction
- Prior exposure to streptokinase or anistreplase (in which case use alteplase)

If there are one or more relative contraindications to thrombolytic therapy, you must weigh the risks and benefits of therapy for the individual before deciding whether or not it should be given

Reference:
Management of acute myocardial infarction. ACC/AHA Task Force. *Circulation* 1990; 82: 664–707.

- **Reinfarction** (prolonged chest pain with fresh ST elevation) should be treated with further thrombolytic therapy. Use alteplase if streptokinase has been given more than 4 days previously.
- **Unstable angina** (angina on minimal exertion or at rest) may occur after infarction: start treatment along standard lines (Chapter

■ **Table 12.5** Thrombolytic therapy: regimens

Regimen	Comment
Streptokinase (SK)	Suitable for the majority of patients. Adjunctive heparin not needed if aspirin is given • **SK 1.5 MU (mega units) given as an IV infusion over 1 hour** • **Aspirin 300 mg PO (chewed), followed by 75–150 mg/day indefinitely**
Alteplase (tPA), standard regimen	Use if the patient has received SK within the previous 4 days to 12 months. Adjunctive heparin and aspirin should be given • **Alteplase 1.5 mg/kg given as an IV infusion over 3 hours** • **Heparin 5000 U IV bolus, followed by a continuous IV infusion to maintain APTT 1.5–2.5 times control (Table 60.10, p. 386) for at least 2 days** • **Aspirin 300 mg PO (chewed), followed by 75–150 mg/day indefinitely**
Alteplase, accelerated (front-loaded) regimen	May be worthwhile in patients aged < 50 with large infarcts presenting within 4 hours who are normotensive (systolic BP < 140 mmHg) – i.e. low risk of haemorrhagic stroke. Adjunctive heparin and aspirin should be given • **Alteplase 15 mg IV bolus, followed by: 0.75 mg/kg (maximum 50 mg) over 30 min; followed by 0.5 mg/kg (maximum 35 mg) over the next 60 min** • **Heparin as above** • **Aspirin as above**

APTT, Activated partial thromboplastin time.

■ **Table 12.6** Thrombolytic therapy: problems

Hypotension during streptokinase infusion

● Usually reversed by elevating the foot of the bed or slowing the infusion

Allergic reaction to streptokinase

● Give chlorpheniramine 10 mg IV and hydrocortisone 100 mg IV (prophylactic treatment not needed)

Oozing from puncture sites

● If venepuncture is necessary, use a 22 gauge (blue) needle and compress the puncture site for 10 min
● Central venous lines should be inserted via an antecubital fossa vein (percutaneously or by cut-down)
● For arterial puncture, use a 23 gauge (orange) needle in the radial or brachial artery and compress the puncture site for at least 10 min

Uncontrollable bleeding

● Stop the infusion
● Transfuse whole fresh blood if available or fresh frozen plasma
● As a last resort, give tranexamic acid 1 g (10 mg/kg) IV over 10 min

Symptomatic bradycardia unresponsive to atropine

● If temporary pacing is required within 24 hours of thrombolytic therapy, the wire should ideally be placed via an antecubital fossa vein. If there is no suitable superficial vein, the options are a cut-down (seek help from a cardiologist if you are not familiar with this) or placement via the femoral vein (p. 319)

13), **and seek expert advice from a cardiologist** about cardiac catheterization.

● **Pericarditis** is a common cause of new chest pain and usually occurs 2–3 days after infarction. The diagnosis is based on the patient's description of the pain: worse on inspiration and eased by sitting forward. A pericardial friction rub is not always heard, and the ECG rarely shows typical ST/T changes of pericarditis. Treat with soluble aspirin 600 mg 6-hourly PO or indomethacin 25–50 mg

■ **Table 12.7** Chest pain after myocardial infarction

Cause	Comment
Infarct	Mild bruised sensation common for 24–36 hours after infarction
Reinfarction	Prolonged pain with fresh ST elevation
Unstable angina	Anginal pain at rest or on minimal exertion
Pericarditis	Pain worse on deep inspiration and eased by leaning forward. Pericardial rub not always heard
Fractured rib	After resuscitation with chest compression. Localized tenderness

■ **Table 12.8** Fever after myocardial infarction

- Due to the infarct itself
- Pericarditis
- Thrombophlebitis at cannula site
- Infection related to a Swan – Ganz catheter or pacing wire
- Deep-vein thrombosis
- Urinary tract infection
- Pneumonia

8-hourly PO until the pain has gone. Echocardiography is not routinely required.

- **Fever** (up to 38°C) and a neutrophil leukocytosis (up to $12-15 \times 10^9/1$) is a common response to infarction, usually with a peak at 3–4 days, but check for other causes (see Table 12.8).
- There are several causes of a **new murmur** which can usually be distinguished on clinical grounds (see Table 12.9). **Echocardiography must be performed urgently: (a)** if the murmur is pansystolic particularly if it is loud or accompanied by a thrill; or **(b)** if there is pulmonary oedema, hypotension or signs of low cardiac output.
- **Ventricular septal rupture** (VSR) may be present on admission

■ Table 12.9 New murmur after myocardial infarction

Cause	Characteristics
Pericarditis	Scratchy, often both systolic and diastolic components. Associated pericardial pain common
Papillary muscle dysfunction	Murmur may occur anywhere in systole or may be pansystolic
Papillary muscle rupture	Pansystolic murmur usually maximal at apex. Pulmonary oedema invariable
Ventricular septal rupture	Pansystolic murmur usually maximal between apex and left sternal edge, and audible to left of thoracic spine (useful in distinguishing from papillary muscle rupture). Faint thrill common. Pulmonary oedema common but not invariable. JVP usually raised

JVP, Jugular venous pressure.

and occurs earlier after thrombolysis (around 3 days). Although VSR usually causes sudden haemodynamic deterioration, with pulmonary oedema and often cardiogenic shock, it may occasionally cause little haemodynamic effect or present late with deteriorating renal function. Echocardiography is needed for accurate differentiation from papillary muscle rupture. Both diagnoses may coexist. **Seek expert advice** from a cardiologist on further management.

5 Prophylactic drug therapy after myocardial infarction.

• If there have been no clinical or radiological signs of heart failure, start a **beta-blocker** (if not contraindicated because of asthma).

• If there have been signs of heart failure, or there is evidence of extensive infarction, start an angiotensin-converting enzyme **(ACE)-inhibitor**.

• The ideal time to start treatment has not been defined but 24 hours after infarction is reasonable.

- If beta-blockade is contraindicated because of asthma, and there is no evidence of heart failure or extensive infarction, consider **verapamil** as an alternative.

6 Patients with an uncomplicated course and suitable home circumstances can be discharged after 5–7 days.

- A predischarge exercise test should be done in patients who have presented with suspected infarction and received thrombolysis but did not have a significant enzyme rise (less than twice the upper limit of normal): if this shows evidence of myocardial ischaemia at a low workload, discuss management with a cardiologist.

- For other patients, arrange an outpatient exercise stress test (if the patient is physically capable of undertaking this): this may be done at 3–4 weeks after infarction and will guide further management.

Haemodynamic problems after myocardial infarction

- **Pulmonary oedema.**
- **Hypotension and low cardiac output.**
- **Arrhythmias and atrioventricular (AV) block.**

Pulmonary oedema

1 Give oxygen.
2 Attach an ECG monitor and correct arrhythmias.
3 If pulmonary oedema is severe, give **diamorphine** 5 mg (2.5 mg if the patient is small or elderly) IV over 3–5 min, with further doses of 2.5 mg every 10–15 min if needed to a maximum of 10 mg. An anti-emetic should also be given (e.g. prochlorperazine 12.5 mg or metoclopramide 10 mg IV).
4 Further treatment depends on the BP.

Systolic BP > 100 mmHg
- Give **frusemide** 40–100 mg IV.

• Give **nitrate** by **IV infusion** (e.g. isosorbide dinitrate 2 mg/hour, increasing by 2 mg/hour every 15–30 min until breathlessness is relieved or systolic BP falls below 100 mmHg or to a maximum of 10 mg/hour), or **buccal administration** (glyceryl trinitrate buccal tablet, 5 mg).

• If there is marked wheeze, give **aminophylline** 250 mg (5 mg/kg) by slow injection or infusion over 10 min watching for ventricular extrasystoles.

Systolic BP < 100 mmHg

Treatment is initially directed at improving the cardiac output and BP (see below).

Hypotension and low cardiac output

(Table 12.10, Fig. 12.2)

1 Give oxygen.

2 Correct arrhythmias.

3 Further treatment depends on whether or not the patient has pulmonary oedema.

No pulmonary oedema

The two possibilities are **hypovolaemia** and **right ventricular infarction**. Hypovolaemia may be due to sweating, vomiting, reduced fluid intake or diuretic therapy.

• **Check the** jugular venous pressure **(JVP)** – low in hypovolaemia and high in right ventricular infarction.

■ **Table 12.10** Signs of a low cardiac output

- **Heart rate:** usually > 100/min
- **Skin:** cool or cold, sweating
- **Mental state:** agitated or confused
- **Urine output:** < 30 ml/hour (< 0.5 mg/kg/hour)
- **Arterial pH:** metabolic acidosis

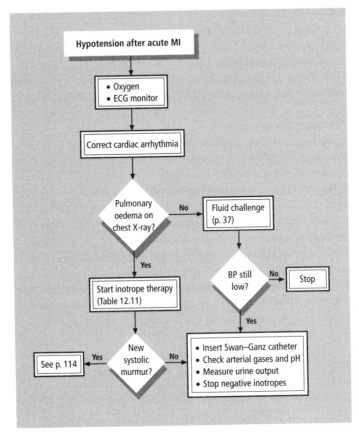

Fig. 12.2 Management of hypotension and low cardiac output after myocardial infarction.

- For both, initial treatment is a **fluid challenge** (p. 37).
- If BP remains low despite fluid challenge, put in a Swan−Ganz catheter − in right ventricular infarction, the right atrial pressure will be high (12−20 mmHg) and equal to or greater than the wedge pressure or pulmonary artery diastolic pressure.

- **Give more fluid if necessary** to raise the wedge pressure/pulmonary artery diastolic pressure to around 15 mmHg.
- **Start dobutamine** if BP remains low despite an adequate left ventricular filling pressure.
- Arrange echocardiography to look for right ventricular infarction (dilated right ventricle with akinesis/dyskinesis of the free wall).

Pulmonary oedema present

- **Start inotropic/vasopressor therapy** (Table 12.11).
- **Arrange urgent echocardiography** to assess left ventricular function and to exclude papillary muscle or ventricular septal rupture.
- **When the patient is stable with an adequate BP, put in a Swan–Ganz catheter.** Measurement of the pulmonary artery diastolic pressure or wedge pressure allows you to titrate therapy to achieve the optimum haemodynamic result. If Swan–Ganz catheterization is not feasible, you must rely on the clinical signs and the chest X-ray to estimate left atrial pressure (Table 12.12).
- **Providing the systolic BP has increased to at least 100 mmHg, start a nitrate infusion**, initially at low dose (e.g. isosorbide dinitrate 2 mg/hour). Adjust the doses of inotrope and nitrate, aiming for a

■ **Table 12.11** Inotropic/vasopressor therapy in myocardial infarction

---

Systolic BP 80–100 mmHg

- **Dobutamine** 5–40 μg/kg/min (p. 381) via a central or peripheral vein. This both increases cardiac output and BP and reduces left atrial pressure

Systolic BP < 80 mmHg

- **Dopamine** 10–40 μg/kg/min via a central vein. At this dose dopamine has a vasoconstrictor effect

If systolic BP remains < 80 mmHg

- **Start noradrenaline** at 0.05 μg/kg/min (p. 375) via a central vein, increasing the dose as required
- **Reduce dopamine** to 2.5 μg/kg/min (renal vasodilator dose (p. 385))

■ **Table 12.12** Acute myocardial infarction: prediction of left atrial pressure from the chest X-ray

Appearances	Likely left atrial pressure (mmHg)
Normal lungs	< 15
Distension of upper lobe veins	15−20
Interstitial pulmonary oedema	20−25
Alveolar pulmonary oedema	> 25

NB: Changes in the chest X-ray may lag several hours behind haemodynamic changes.

pulmonary artery (PA) diastolic/wedge pressure of 15−20 mmHg with a systolic BP of > 100 mmHg.
● Diuretics are ineffective in patients with cardiogenic shock, but can be used once the cardiac output has increased (as shown by improvement in the patient's mental state and skin perfusion).

Arrhythmias and atrioventricular block

Bradyarrhythmias and atrioventricular block
● For details of diagnosis and management, see Chapter 2, p. 9.
● Atropine 0.6−1.2 mg IV is the first-line treatment of symptomatic bradycardia.
● Generally accepted indications for temporary pacing (p. 332) are given in Table 12.13: discuss the case with a cardiologist if you are uncertain about the need for pacing.

Tachyarrhythmias
For details of diagnosis and management, see Chapter 2, p. 9. Tachyarrhythmias are managed along standard lines bearing in mind the following points:
● **Hypokalaemia, hypoxia, acidosis and anxiety predispose to arrhythmias and should be corrected.** In patients with significant arrhythmias, plasma potassium should be kept at 4−5 mmol/l.

■ **Table 12.13** Indications for temporary pacing in acute myocardial infarction

- Asystole (after restoration of spontaneous rhythm)
- Complete heart block
- Right bundle branch block with new left anterior hemiblock or left posterior hemiblock*
- New left bundle branch block
- Mobitz type II second-degree AV block
- Mobitz type I (Wenckebach) second-degree AV block with hypotension not responsive to atropine
- Sinus bradycardia with hypotension or recurrent sinus pauses not responsive to atropine
- Atrial or ventricular overdrive pacing for recurrent ventricular tachycardia (seek advice from a cardiologist)

* Left anterior hemiblock gives left-axis deviation (S wave > R in lead II); left posterior hemiblock gives right-axis deviation (S wave > R in lead I).
Reference:
Management of acute myocardial infarction. ACC/AHA Task Force. *Circulation* 1990; 82: 664–707.

- **Accelerated idioventricular rhythm** (regular broad-complex rhythm at a rate < 120/min) does not need treatment.
- **Regular broad-complex tachycardia (rate > 120/min) after infarction is almost always ventricular tachycardia (VT)** rather than supraventricular tachycardia (SVT) with aberrant conduction (p. 9): if there is any doubt, assume it is VT. The safest treatment is lignocaine or synchronized DC shock. **Verapamil can cause severe hypotension (and death) if given for VT.**

Appendix 1

- Peak enzyme levels are usually higher and reached earlier after thrombolysis with reperfusion.
- Raised CK-MB levels may also occur in the following: myocarditis, cardiac trauma, hypothermia, subarachnoid haemorrhage and renal failure.

■ **Table 12.14** Enzyme changes after myocardial infarction

Enzyme	Rises (hours)	Peaks	Returns to normal (days)
CK	4−8	12−24 hours	3−4
CK-MB	4−8	12−20 hours	2−3
AST	8−12	18−36 hours	3−4
LDH	8−12	3−6 days	8−14

CK, Creatine kinase; CK-MB, MB isoenzyme of creatine kinase; AST, aspartate transaminase (glutamic oxaloacetic transaminase); LDH, lactic dehydrogenase.

Reference:
Lee TH, Goldman L. Serum enzyme assays in the diagnosis of acute myocardial infarction. Recommendations based on a quantitative analysis. *Ann Intern Med* 1986; 105: 221−33.

13 Unstable angina

- Unstable angina is a term used to describe the clinical syndromes that range in severity from a change in the pattern of exertional angina to pre-infarction angina with prolonged rest pain.
- Consider the diagnosis in any patient with **chest pain at rest but without ST elevation on the ECG**.

Priorities

1 **Take a careful history of the chest pain** (Table 4.2, p. 44), **examine the patient and record an ECG. Give sublingual nitrate if there is pain at rest.**

- Features supporting a diagnosis of unstable angina are given in Table 13.1. If none of these is present, unstable angina is unlikely and other causes of chest pain must be pursued.

2 **On the basis of your clinical assessment and the ECG appearances, patients with unstable angina can be assigned to one of three groups (Table 13.2) which determine management.**

3 **Further investigations are listed in Table 13.3.**

Low-risk patients

- Send home on treatment with aspirin, a beta-blocker or calcium antagonist, and sublingual nitrate as required (Table 13.4).
- Tell the patient to return to hospital if symptoms worsen.
- Arrange for follow-up by the GP within 3 days.
- Arrange outpatient follow-up after an exercise test.

Medium-risk patients

- Admit to the general ward.
- Heparin is not required as initial treatment. Start aspirin and a beta-blocker or calcium antagonist (see Table 13.4).
- If chest pain recurs at rest, manage as high risk.

■ **Table 13.1** Chest pain: features supporting a diagnosis of unstable angina

- Preceding similar exertional chest pain
- Relief of chest pain with nitrate
- Known coronary artery disease (previous myocardial infarction or angiographically proven)
- Risk factors for coronary artery disease (multiple factors or single major factor such as familial hypercholesterolaemia)
- Abnormal ECG with ST depression and/or T-wave inversion

■ **Table 13.2** Stratification of patients with unstable angina

Clinical group	Characteristics
Low risk	New onset or worsening exertional angina No episodes of severe, prolonged (> 20 min) or rest pain in the preceding 2 weeks
Medium risk	One or more episodes of severe, prolonged or rest pain in the preceding 2 weeks No haemodynamic abnormalities No ECG abnormalities not known to be old
High risk	One or more of the following features: **(a)** ongoing chest pain: **(b)** recent myocardial infarction: **(c)** pulmonary oedema: **(d)** new or worsening mitral regurgitation: **(e)** hypotension: or **(f)** new ST/T wave abnormalities

■ **Table 13.3** Investigation in unstable angina

- **ECG** on admission, daily for 3 days and if pain recurs
- **Chest X-ray**
- **Cardiac enzymes** on admission, daily for 2 days and if pain recurs
- **Urea, sodium and potassium**
- **Blood glucose**
- **Full blood count** (to exclude anaemia)
- **Cholesterol**

■ Table 13.4 Drug therapy in unstable angina

Drug	Regimen
Aspirin	300 mg PO (chewed) followed by 150 mg daily
Beta-blocker	Atenolol 50–100 mg/day PO or Metoprolol 50–100 mg 8- to 12-hourly PO
Calcium antagonist	If beta-blockade is contraindicated because of heart failure, asthma or chronic airflow limitation Diltiazem 60–120 mg 8-hourly PO
Heparin	5000 U IV over 5 min, followed by an infusion to maintain APTT 1.5–2.5 × control (p. 386)
Nitrate	Either by IV or buccal route IV: isosorbide dinitrate 2 mg/hour, increasing by 2 mg/ hour every 15–30 min until pain is relieved or systolic BP falls below 100 mmHg or to a maximum of 10 mg/hour Buccal: glyceryl trinitrate (buccal tablet), 5 mg 6-hourly

APTT, Activated partial thromboplastin time.

High-risk patients

- Admit to the cardiac care unit.
- If there is chest pain at rest or pulmonary oedema, give nitrate by IV infusion or buccal administration (see Table 13.4).
- Start aspirin, heparin and a beta-blocker or calcium antagonist.

Further management (Fig. 13.1)

Medium-risk patients

- Bed rest for 12–24 hours followed by a programme of mobilization.
- If there is no recurrence of chest pain, perform an exercise stress test before discharge.

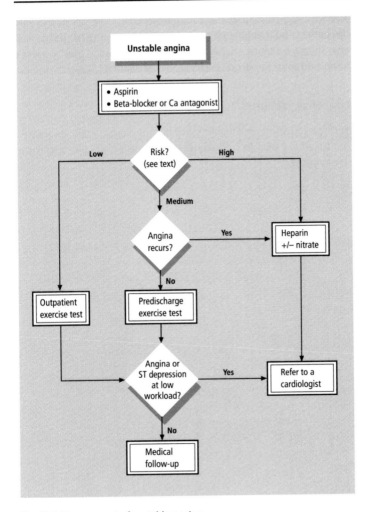

Fig. 13.1 Management of unstable angina.

• Discuss further management with a cardiologist before discharging the patient: **(a)** if angina occurs on mobilisation; or **(b)** if the exercise test shows evidence of myocardial ischaemia at a low workload (under 6 min of the Bruce protocol, or equivalent).

High-risk patients

• Discuss further management with a cardiologist: cardiac catheterization with a view to coronary revascularization will be indicated in the majority.

14 Aortic dissection

Consider the diagnosis in any patient with **chest or upper abdominal pain**, especially if:

- the pain was of **instantaneous onset**; or
- the pain **radiated along the course of the aorta or its major branches**; or
- there are **associated neurological symptoms** (e.g. syncope, stroke, leg weakness); or
- the patient is at increased risk of dissection because of **hypertension, Marfan syndrome or pregnancy.**

Aortic dissection is classified as **proximal** (ascending aorta involved) or **distal** (ascending aorta not involved) (Fig. 14.1, Table 14.1).

Priorities

1 Relieve pain with diamorphine 5 mg IV (in small or elderly people 2.5 mg) with further doses every 15 min as required. Complete your clinical assessment (Table 14.2).

2 Obtain an ECG and chest X-ray.
- The ECG is principally of use in assessing the likelihood of acute myocardial infarction (p. 107) (aortic dissection can rarely involve the coronary arteries and cause infarction).
- The chest X-ray is often normal particularly in dissection involving only the ascending aorta (Table 14.3).

3 The working diagnosis is aortic dissection if:
- the pain was of instantaneous onset, and no alternative diagnosis can be made; **or**
- one or more major pulses is absent or asymmetric; **or**
- there is aortic regurgitation; **or**
- the chest X-ray shows a widened mediastinum.

4 If the diagnosis is secure, start hypotensive therapy (Table 14.4) and arrange immediate transfer to a cardiothoracic unit.

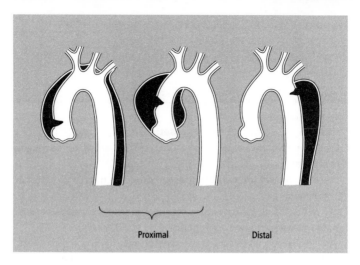

Fig. 14.1 Classification of aortic dissection.

■ **Table 14.1** Classification of aortic dissection

Feature	Proximal	Distal
Site of tear in aortic intima	Just above aortic valve	Just beyond origin of left subclavian artery
Origin of pain	Retrosternal	Interscapular
Pulse abnormalities	Present in 50%	Present in 15%
Aortic regurgitation	Present in 50%	Present in 10%*
Pericardial effusion	Present in 20%	Not found
Common misdiagnosis	Myocardial infarction	Myocardial infarction
		Acute abdomen
Management	Surgical	Medical

* Aortic regurgitation may be present in distal aortic dissection due to preexisting aortic root dilatation.

■ **Table 14.2** Examination in suspected aortic dissection

- **BP in both arms** (the difference in systolic pressure is normally < 15 mmHg)
- **Signs of tamponade** (raised JVP/pulsus paradoxus) (if found, immediately contact a cardiothoracic surgeon)
- **Peripheral pulses**
- **Early diastolic murmur of aortic regurgitation** (listen with the patient leaning forward in expiration)
- **Limb power, tendon reflexes and plantar responses**

JVP, Jugular venous pressure.

■ **Table 14.3** Chest X-ray findings in aortic dissection

Radiological feature	Percentage
Abnormal knuckle (widening/double lumen)	66
Irregular aortic contour	38
Discrepancy in diameter of ascending and descending aorta	34
Pleural effusion	27
Mediastinal widening	11
Displacement of calcified intima	7
Normal PA and left lateral films	18

Reference:
Earnest F *et al.* Roentgenographic findings in thoracic aortic dissection. *Mayo Clin Proc* 1979; 54: 43–50.

5 For other patients, definitive investigation is needed – for example computed tomography (CT) scan with contrast or **transoesophageal echocardiography (TOE)** (Table 14.4) as available.

Further management of confirmed aortic dissection

1 Transfer the patient to an intensive therapy unit or cardiac care unit and start treatment to reduce the BP (Table 14.4).

- Make sure adequate analgesia has been given.

■ **Table 14.4** Investigation of suspected aortic dissection

Investigation	Comment
Transthoracic echocardiography	Useful screening test, but sensitivity only 50% for proximal dissection and 30% for distal dissection. Gives information about pericardial effusion, aortic regurgitation and left ventricular (LV) function
Transoesophageal echocardiography (TOE)	Excellent sensitivity for proximal and distal dissection. Specificity suboptimal in proximal dissection — plaque formation or echo reverberations in ectatic vessel may give false positive results. Major advantage over CT or MRI is that it can be performed rapidly at the bedside
Computed tomography with contrast (CT)	More widely available in district general hospitals than TOE or MRI. Sensitivity slightly lower than TOE. Gives no information about aortic regurgitation or LV function
Magnetic resonance imaging (MRI)	Excellent sensitivity, and higher specificity than TOE or CT. Not practical in patients who are ventilated or who require extensive monitoring

High sensitivity — low false negative rate.
High specificity — low false positive rate.

- BP should be monitored continuously with an intra-arterial line if you use nitroprusside or trimetaphan.
- Put in a urinary catheter to monitor urine output.
- Aim to reduce systolic BP to 100–120 mmHg, providing the urine output remains > 30 ml/hour.

2 Discuss management with a cardiologist. Patients with **proximal dissection** who are candidates for surgery will be transferred urgently for this. Patients with **distal dissection** should be managed medically, and weaned on to oral hypotensive therapy. Surgery is indicated for persistent or recurrent pain, occlusion of a major artery or high risk of rupture (e.g. Marfan syndrome).

■ **Table 14.5** Options for hypotensive therapy for acute aortic dissection

1 Labetolol infusion

- Make up a solution of 1 mg/ml by diluting the contents of 2 ampoules (200 mg) to 200 ml with normal saline or dextrose 5%
- Start the infusion at 0.25 mg/min (15 ml/hour) and increase it every 15 min as necessary

2 Nitroprusside plus propranolol

Nitroprusside infusion (NB: continuous intra-arterial pressure monitoring needed)

- Make up a solution of 100 μg/ml by adding 50 mg to 500 ml dextrose 5%
- Start the infusion at 6 ml/hour (10 μg/min) and increase it by steps of 10 μg/min every 5 min as necessary to a maximum dose of 75 μg/min

Propranolol

- Give 0.1 mg/kg IV every 4–6 hours

3 Trimetaphan infusion (NB: continuous intra-arterial pressure monitoring needed)

- This should be used if there are contraindications to beta-blockade such as airways obstruction or congestive heart failure
- Make up a solution of 10 mg/ml by diluting the contents of 2 ampoules (500 mg) to 50 ml with normal saline or dextrose 5%
- Start the infusion at 6 ml/hour (1 mg/min) and increase the infusion rate every 15 min as necessary

15 Severe hypertension

- Defined by a diastolic BP > 120 mmHg.
- **Emergency IV therapy is rarely required and is potentially danger-ous.** Abrupt reduction of BP may cause stroke, myocardial infarction or renal failure.

Priorities

1 **Check BP yourself.** Look for evidence of an underlying cause (Table 15.1). **Examine the fundi.** Investigations needed urgently are given in Table 15.2.

2 The following **are indications for emergency treatment:**
- left ventricular failure with alveolar pulmonary oedema;
- hypertensive encephalopathy (see below);
- acute aortic dissection.

3 **If emergency treatment is needed transfer the patient to the intensive-therapy unit.** Consider the need for an intra-arterial line to allow continuous monitoring of the BP and a urinary catheter to monitor urine output.

4 Give **frusemide** 40−80 mg IV if there is left ventricular failure or encephalopathy.

5 Start **IV antihypertensive therapy** (Table 15.3).

Further management

1 **Admit the patient if there is:**
- papilloedema, retinal haemorrhages or exudates;
- renal failure;
- interstitial pulmonary oedema;
- diastolic BP > 130 mmHg.

2 **Start oral therapy** (Table 15.4). Recheck the BP every 30 min. If the

■ **Table 15.1** Causes of secondary hypertension

Cause	Comment
Drugs	Corticosteroids, carbenoxolone, oral contraceptives
Coarctation of the aorta	Radiofemoral delay
Renal artery stenosis	Abdominal bruit may be heard Peripheral arterial disease
Renal disease	Raised urea and creatinine, abnormal urinalysis or urinary sediment on microscopy
Phaeochromocytoma	Paroxysmal headache, sweating, or palpitation
Primary hyperaldosteronism (Conn syndrome)	Bilateral adrenal hyperplasia or adrenal tumour Hypokalaemia
Cushing syndrome	Corticosteroid therapy, pituitary or adrenal tumour Truncal obesity, thin skin with purple abdominal striae, proximal myopathy

■ **Table 15.2** Urgent investigation of the patient with severe hypertension

- Urea, sodium and potassium
- Urinalysis (plus urine microscopy if abnormal)
- Chest X-ray
- ECG

diastolic BP is unchanged after 4 hours, repeat the dose or add another drug.

3 Seek expert advice from a nephrologist if there is:
- evidence of acute glomerulonephritis (> 2+ proteinuria and/or red-cell casts in the urine) (p. 248);
- acute renal failure (Chapter 36).

■ **Table 15.3** IV therapy for hypertensive emergencies: aim to reduce diastolic BP to 100–110 mmHg within 1 hour

Options:

1 Labetalol – the treatment of choice if there is **aortic dissection or suspected phaeochromocytoma**; avoid in left ventricular failure
 • Make up a solution of 1 mg/ml by diluting the contents of 2 ampoules (200 mg) to 200 ml with normal saline or dextrose 5%
 • Start the infusion at 0.25 mg/min (15 ml/hour) and increase it every 15 min to a maximum dose of 200 mg/min (high doses may be needed in phaeochromocytoma)

2 Nitroprusside – the treatment of choice if there is **severe left ventricular failure or hypertensive encephalopathy**
 • Should not be used without continuous intra-arterial pressure monitoring
 • Make up a solution of 100 μg/ml by adding 50 mg to 500 ml dextrose 5%
 • Start the infusion at 6 ml/hour (10 μg/min) and increase it by steps of 10 μg/min every 5 min to a maximum dose of 75 μg/min.

■ **Table 15.4** Initial oral therapy for severe hypertension: aim to reduce diastolic BP to around 110 mmHg over the first 24 hours

Clinical features	Drug therapy
Interstitial pulmonary oedema	**Frusemide** 20 mg (higher doses will be necessary in patients with impaired renal function) plus **nifedipine**, 10–20 mg 8-hourly
Phaeochromocytoma suspected	**Labetalol** 100–200 mg 12-hourly
Beta-blockers contraindicated	**Nifedipine** 10–20 mg 8-hourly or **clonidine** 100–200 μg 8-hourly or **hydralazine** 25–50 mg 8-hourly
Other patients	**Atenolol** 50–100 mg once daily or **any of the above**

NB: avoid angiotensin-converting enzyme (ACE)-inhibitors as initial treatment because of unpredictable first-dose hypotension.

■ **Table 15.5** Clinical features of hypertensive encephalopathy

Early features	• Headache
	• Nausea and vomiting
	• Confusional state
	• Retinal haemorrhages, exudates or papilloedema
Late features	• Focal neurological signs
	• Fits
	• Coma

Problems

Hypertensive encephalopathy, subarachnoid haemorrhage or stroke?

• These may be difficult to distinguish clinically. Hypertensive encephalopathy (Table 15.5) is favoured by: **(a)** gradual onset of symptoms; **(b)** focal neurological signs absent, or appearing late.

• If there is diagnostic doubt, a computed tomography (CT) scan should be obtained to exclude cerebral or subarachnoid haemorrhage before starting IV therapy (see Table 15.3).

Recent stroke

• Rapid lowering of the BP may worsen the neurological deficit. Treat if systolic BP > 200 mmHg or diastolic BP > 120 mmHg after 48 hours (for treatment see Table 15.4).

16 Pulmonary oedema

Causes

• **High pulmonary capillary pressure** from cardiac disease or fluid overload (overtransfusion, renal failure).

• **Increased pulmonary capillary permeability** – the acute respiratory distress syndrome (ARDS) or 'shock lung' (Appendix 1).

Priorities

1 **Give oxygen 35–60%.** Pulse oximetry may be unreliable due to peripheral vasoconstriction, and arterial blood gases should be checked.

2 **Check the BP and pulse and listen to the heart and lungs.**
   • If there is any diagnostic doubt, obtain a chest X-ray before starting drug treatment. Inspiratory crackles are not always present; wheeze is common and may lead to the misdiagnosis of asthma.

3 **Attach an ECG monitor and treat arrhythmias** (Chapter 2).

4 **Put in a peripheral IV cannula and give the following drugs:**
   • **diamorphine** 2.5–5.0 mg (or morphine 5.0–10.0 mg) by slow IV injection;
   • **frusemide** 40–80 mg IV;
   • **if systolic BP is >90 mmHg, nitrate** sublingually (glyceryl trinitrate spray 2 puffs) or buccally (glyceryl trinitrate 2 mg or 5 mg buccal tablet).

5 **If pulmonary oedema is due to overtransfusion**, venesect using a large-bore cannula or a blood-donation set.

6 **Investigations required urgently** are given in Table 16.1.

7 **Has the patient got ARDS** rather than cardiogenic pulmonary oedema (Table 16.2)? The management of ARDS is outlined in Appendix 1.

8 **Has the patient got renal failure?** In patients with a blood urea

■ **Table 16.1** Urgent investigation in pulmonary oedema

● **ECG** (? arrhythmia; ? evidence of infarction or other cardiac disease, e.g. left ventricular hypertrophy, left bundle branch block)

● **Chest X-ray** (to confirm the clinical diagnosis and exclude other causes of breathlessness – effusion, pneumothorax, pneumonia)

● **Arterial blood gases** and pH (if not improving within 30 min)

● **Urea, sodium and potassium**

● **Echocardiogram** (if the cause of pulmonary oedema is uncertain)

■ **Table 16.2** When to suspect acute respiratory distress syndrome rather than cardiogenic pulmonary oedema

● **The patient is at risk of ARDS:** sepsis, major trauma, major surgery, acute pancreatitis and opiate poisoning are the most important predisposing factors
● **Normal ECG**
● **Chest X-ray shows diffuse bilateral shadowing** (often sparing the costophrenic angles), but **without cardiomegaly or distension of upper-lobe pulmonary veins**

> 20 mmol/1, conventional doses of frusemide are often ineffective.
● Try a frusemide infusion (30–60 mg/hour).
● If this fails, dialysis will be needed. In extreme circumstances, venesect 500 ml while this is being arranged.

Further management of cardiogenic pulmonary oedema

Further drug therapy depends on the blood pressure

1 **Systolic BP > 100 mmHg.**
● Give another dose of frusemide 40–80 mg IV.

- Start a **nitrate infusion** (p. 116). If the patient remains breathless, increase the infusion rate every 15–30 min providing systolic BP is > 100 mmHg.

2 **Systolic BP 80–100 mmHg.**

- Start a **dobutamine infusion** at a dose of 5 µg/kg/min (p. 381). Increase the dose by 2.5 µg/kg/min every 10 min until systolic BP is > 100 mmHg or a maximum dose of 20 µg/kg/min has been reached.

- A nitrate infusion can be added if systolic BP is maintained at > 100 mmHg.

3 **Systolic BP < 80 mmHg (cardiogenic shock).**

- Systolic BP must be rapidly increased to > 90 mmHg to maintain coronary, cerebral and renal perfusion.

- Give adrenaline 0.5–1 mg by slow IV injection (5–10 ml of 1 in 10 000 solution) via a central or large antecubital vein.

- Start a dopamine infusion at 10 µg/kg/min. Increase the dose by 5 µg/kg/min every 15 min until systolic BP is > 100 mmHg. If systolic BP remains < 90 mmHg despite dopamine 20 µg/kg/min, use noradrenaline instead (p. 374).

Check arterial gases and pH

- Increase the inspired oxygen concentration if necessary to maintain Pa_{O_2} around 10 kPa.

- Continous positive airway pressure delivered through a tight-fitting facemask can improve oxygenation and reduce the need for mechanical ventilation, and may be helpful in patients with severe

■ **Table 16.3** Indications for Swan–Ganz catheterization in the patient with pulmonary oedema

- **Suspected ARDS** (Tables 16.2 and 16.6)
- **Exclusion of ventricular septal rupture** in the patient with pulmonary oedema and a systolic murmur after myocardial infarction if echocardiography is not available (p. 329)
- **Associated hypotension** requiring treatment with an inotrope

pulmonary oedema: discuss this with a chest physician or anaesthetist.

- Mechanical ventilation is indicated if Pao_2 is < 8 kPa despite 60% oxygen, or $Paco_2$ is rising, if recovery from the underlying cause is possible.
- If arterial pH is less than 7.2, infuse 50 mmol of sodium bicarbonate (50 ml of 8.4% solution) over 15 min (severe metabolic acidosis has a negative inotropic effect and facilitates ventricular arrhythmias).

Systolic BP < 90 mmHg or no urine passed after 1 hour?

- Put in a urinary catheter.
- The urine output is a good guide to the cardiac output and should ideally be > 30 ml/hour (> 0.5 ml/kg/hour).

Put in a Swan–Ganz catheter if indicated (Table 16.3)

- Adjust the doses of inotrope and nitrate, aiming for a pulmonary artery (PA) diastolic/wedge pressure of 15–20 mmHg with a systolic BP > 100 mmHg.

Decide what has caused or precipitated the attack
(Tables 16.4 and 16.5)

- Discuss further management with a cardiologist if you suspect valvular disease or ventricular septal rupture (for which urgent surgery may be needed).
- Stop drugs with a negative inotropic effect.

■ **Table 16.4** Causes of cardiogenic pulmonary oedema 'out of the blue'

- Arrhythmia with underlying LV or valvular disease
- Painless myocardial infarction
- Acute myocarditis
- Acute aortic regurgitation (aortic dissection, bacterial endocarditis)
- Acute mitral regurgitation (ruptured chordae or papillary muscle) (p. 114)
- Ventricular septal rupture after myocardial infarction (p. 114)
- Severe mitral stenosis
- Severe aortic stenosis
- Pulmonary oedema complicating acute central nervous system disease (e.g. subarachnoid haemorrhage)
- Left atrial myxoma

LV, Left ventricular.

■ **Table 16.5** Precipitants of pulmonary oedema in patients with previously stable valvular or left ventricular disease

- Myocardial infarction
- Arrhythmia (the onset of atrial fibrillation is a common precipitant of pulmonary oedema in patients with severe mitral or aortic stenosis)
- Drugs with a negative inotropic effect (e.g. beta-blockers)
- Poor compliance with diuretic therapy
- Drugs causing fluid retention (e.g. NSAIDs, steroids)
- Excessive IV fluid or blood (e.g. given peri-operatively or after GI bleeding)

NSAIDs, Non-steroidal anti-inflammatory drugs; GI, gastrointestinal.

Appendix 1: acute respiratory distress syndrome

ARDS is the result of pulmonary endothelial damage, usually occurring as part of multiple organ failure. Patients with suspected ARDS (Table 16.6) should be referred early to the ITU. The key elements in management are:

■ **Table 16.6** Diagnostic criteria for acute respiratory distress syndrome

• **Antecedent history of precipitating condition** (e.g. sepsis, major trauma, major surgery, acute pancreatitis, opiate poisoning)
• **Refractory hypoxaemia** ($Pao_2 < 8$ kPa (60 mmHg), Fio_2 40%;
arterial : alveolar oxygen-tension ratio < 0.25)
• **Bilateral pulmonary infiltrates** on chest X-ray
• **Pulmonary artery wedge pressure $< 15-18$ mmHg** (with normal colloid oncotic pressure)
• **Total thoracic compliance < 30 ml/cm water**

Reference:
Macnaughton PD, Evans TW. Management of adult respiratory distress syndrome. *Lancet* 1992; 339: 469–72.

Maintenance of oxygenation

• Keep Pao_2 9–11 kPa by adjusting the inspired oxygen concentration (Fio_2). Ventilation will be needed if Pao_2 is < 7 kPa despite Fio_2 60%.
• Haemoglobin should be kept around 10 g/dl (to give the optimum balance between oxygen carrying capacity and blood viscosity).
• Oxygen delivery (Do_2) (see Table 52.4, p. 331) may be increased by fluid loading and dobutamine infusion.

Fluid balance

• Pulmonary artery wedge pressure should be kept 10–15 mmHg.
• Renal failure is commonly associated with ARDS and may be managed by haemofiltration.

Prevention and treatment of sepsis

• Sepsis is a common cause and complication of ARDS.
• Enteral feeding may carry a lower risk of pulmonary infection than parenteral nutrition.
• Culture blood, tracheobronchial aspirate and urine daily. Treat presumed infection with broad-spectrum antibiotic therapy.

Prevention of gastric stress ulceration

• Sucralfate 1 g 6-hourly by nasogastric tube (associated with a lower incidence of pulmonary infection than H_2-receptor blockers).

Drug therapy in acute lung injury

• There is no firm evidence that high-dose corticosteroid affects the course of established ARDS and it should not be given.
• Other therapies (e.g. surfactant) are experimental.

17 Pericarditis

Consider the diagnosis in any patient with:
- **central chest pain that is worse on inspiration and relieved by sitting forward;**
- **pericardial friction rub** (pericarditis may be painless);
- **unexplained enlargement of the cardiac shadow on the chest X-ray** (reflecting a pericardial effusion).

Causes of pericarditis are given in Table 17.1.

Priorities

1 Relieve pain: an NSAID is usually sufficient (e.g. indomethacin 25–50 mg 8-hourly PO). Severe pain may require an opiate.

2 Obtain an ECG. The diagnosis of pericarditis is based on the clinical features supported by the ECG (Table 17.2). Note the following points.

- The ECG is rarely helpful in pericarditis after myocardial infarction (the commonest cause of pericarditis seen in hospital).
- The changes on the initial ECG may be impossible to distinguish from those of acute myocardial infarction. If there is diagnostic doubt, thrombolytic therapy must not be given.
- The ECG may be normal in around 10% of patients with pericarditis.

3 Is there evidence of cardiac tamponade: hypotension or breathlessness associated with raised jugular venous pressure (JVP) and pulsus paradoxus? If so:
- **obtain an echocardiogram** urgently;
- consider **pericardiocentesis** if a significant effusion is confirmed (echo separation > 2 cm) (p. 341).

4 Further investigations (Table 17.3) are directed at establishing the underlying cause.

■ **Table 17.1** Causes of pericarditis

- Idiopathic (i.e. no underlying cause found)
- Infectious diseases (viral, bacterial, fungal and tuberculous)
- Acute myocardial infarction
- Collagen disease, e.g. SLE
- Uraemia
- Pericardial surgery, trauma or irradiation
- Dressler syndrome and postcardiotomy syndrome
- Drugs, e.g. procainamide, hydralazine
- Neoplastic diseases (most commonly carcinoma of the bronchus or breast)
- Myxoedema

SLE, Systemic lupus erythematosus.

■ **Table 17.2** The ECG in pericarditis compared with myocardial infarction and early repolarization

ECG Feature	Myocardial infarction	Pericarditis
• ST morphology	Usually convex	Usually concave
• Distribution	Inferior, anterior or lateral patterns	Commonly both limb and chest leads
• Q waves	Usual	Never occur
• ST and T wave evolution	Uniform in all affected leads	Various stages occur concurrently
• QT prolongation	May occur	Does not occur

ECG Feature	Early repolarization	Pericarditis
• ST morphology	Concave	Concave
• Leads showing ST elevation	Commonly septal, rarely limb	Both limb and chest
• ST elevation V6	Uncommon	Common
• ST depression V1	Rare	Common
• PR depression in precordial leads	Rare	Common

References:

Goldberger AL. *Myocardial infarction: electrocardiac differential diagnosis.* CV Mosby, 1975.

Spodick DH. Differential characteristics of the electrocardiogram in early repolarisation and acute pericarditis. *N Engl J Med* 1976; 295: 523–6.

■ **Table 17.3** Investigation in suspected pericarditis

- Chest X-ray – ? enlarged cardiac shadow, ? interstitial oedema, ? consolidation
- ECG (see Table 17.2)
- Cardiac enzyme series if myocardial infarction possible (for later analysis; p. 121)
- Full blood count
- ESR
- Urea, sodium and potassium
- Echocardiogram (if cardiac tamponade suspected or cardiac shadow enlarged – ? effusion or myocarditis)
- Blood for viral serology (for later analysis)
- Blood culture (if suspected bacterial infection)
- Autoantibody screen (for later analysis)

ESR, Erythrocyte sedimentation rate.

Further management

Idiopathic or presumed viral pericarditis

- Is the likely cause of pericarditis in young and otherwise healthy adults, and may be preceded by a 'flu-like illness'.
- Is usually a self-limiting illness lasting 1–3 weeks.
- Treat with soluble aspirin 600 mg 6-hourly PO or indomethacin 25–50 mg 8-hourly PO until the pain has gone.
- Recurrent pericarditis may occur in 15–40% of patients.

Pericarditis after myocardial infarction

- Is a common cause of new chest pain, occurring in 10–15% of patients, usually 2–3 days after infarction.
- A pericardial rub is not always heard, and the ECG rarely shows typical ST/T changes of pericarditis.

- Treat with soluble aspirin 600 mg 6-hourly PO or indomethacin 25–50 mg 8-hourly PO until the pain has gone.
- Echocardiography is not routinely required.

Dressler syndrome/postcardiotomy syndrome

- This is an acute illness with fever, pleuritis and pericarditis.
- Occurs in < 1% of patients after myocardial infarction, but around 15% of patients after cardiac surgery, usually 2–4 weeks after the event (range 1 week to 3 months).
- ECG may show typical changes of pericarditis or non-specific ST/T abnormalities.
- Chest X-ray may show an enlarged cardiac silhouette (due to pericardial effusion), bilateral pleural effusions, and transient pulmonary infiltrates.
- The ESR is raised (often > 70 mm/hour).
- An echocardiogram should be obtained to determine the presence and size of pericardial effusion.
- Treat with soluble aspirin 600 mg 6-hourly PO or indomethacin 25–50 mg 8-hourly PO until the pain has gone.
- Prednisolone (initially 40 mg daily PO, tapered off over 1 month) can be given if pain persists > 48 hours despite treatment with aspirin or a non-steroidal anti-inflammatory drug (NSAID).

Bacterial pericarditis

- Is usually due to contiguous spread of intrathoracic infection (e.g. following thoracic surgery or trauma, or complicating bacterial pneumonia).
- If suspected, start antibiotic therapy after taking blood cultures: **flucloxacillin** 1 g 6-hourly IV plus **gentamicin** IV (p. 84).
- Obtain an echocardiogram to look for an effusion or evidence of endocarditis.
- Perform pericardiocentesis if there is an effusion large enough to be drained safely (e.g. echo-free space > 2 cm) (p. 341). Send fluid for cell count, Gram stain and culture. Consider tuberculous or fungal

infection if the effusion is purulent but no organisms are seen on Gram stain.

- Discuss further management with a cardiologist.

18 Cardiac tamponade

Consider cardiac tamponade in any patient with **hypotension or breathlessness associated with**:
- **raised jugular venous pressure (JVP)**; and
- **pulsus paradoxus (Table 18.1)**.

Suspect especially after the insertion of a central line or in the presence of predisposing conditions (Table 18.2).

Priorities

1 Give oxygen, attach an ECG monitor and put in a peripheral venous cannula.

2 **Obtain an ECG and chest X-ray** to exclude other causes of hypotension or breathlessness (Table 18.3).

3 **Obtain an echocardiogram** to confirm the presence of a pericardial effusion, to exclude biventricular failure and to check that there is sufficient fluid along the chosen needle path.

4 Perform **pericardiocentesis** immediately if a significant effusion is present (echo separation >2 cm) (p. 341). **Seek expert advice first in the following circumstances**:
- signs of tamponade but small effusion (echo separation <2 cm);
- effusion with dilated left ventricle (pericardiocentesis may lead to further ventricular dilatation).

5 If pericardiocentesis cannot be performed immediately and systolic BP is <90 mmHg, treat with IV colloid or blood together with an infusion of dopamine or noradrenaline (p. 374) via a central line.

Further management

This is directed at the underlying cause (see Table 18.2).
- Patients with malignant effusions will usually require further in-

■ **Table 18.1** Pulsus paradoxus

1 Defined as a fall in systolic BP $> 10\,mmHg$ on inspiration. May occur in cardiac tamponade, acute severe asthma and right ventricular failure
2 Severe pulsus paradoxus can be detected by palpation of the femoral or brachial pulses. It can be quantified as follows:
- Inflate the blood pressure cuff above systolic BP
- Slowly deflate the cuff, watching the chest, and note the pressure at which sounds are first heard in expiration
- Continue deflating the cuff and note the pressure at which sounds are heard thoughout expiration and inspiration

■ **Table 18.2** Causes of cardiac tamponade

Cause	Percentage
Malignant disease (most commonly carcinoma of the bronchus or breast)	32
Idiopathic pericarditis	14
Uraemia	9
Acute myocardial infarction (receiving heparin)	9
Diagnostic procedures with cardiac perforation	7.5
Bacterial pericarditis	7.5
Tuberculous pericarditis	5
Radiation	4
Myxoedema	4
Aortic dissection	4
Postcardiotomy syndrome	2
Systemic lupus erythematosus	2
Cardiomyopathy (receiving anticoagulants)	2

Reference:
Guberman BA *et al.* Cardiac tamponade in medical patients. *Circulation* 1981; 64: 633–40.

tervention to prevent recurrent tamponade, e.g. radiotherapy or creation of a pericardial window.
- Antibiotic therapy for bacterial pericarditis is given on p. 146.

■ **Table 18.3** Causes of hypotension with raised jugular venous pressure

- Cardiac tamponade
- Severe biventricular failure
- Pulmonary embolism (p. 155)
- Right ventricular infarction (p. 117)
- Severe pulmonary heart disease
- Acute severe asthma (p. 160)
- Tension pneumothorax (p. 179)

19 Deep-vein thrombosis

- Deep-vein thrombosis cannot reliably be confirmed or excluded on clinical grounds. Venography is the most widely available diagnostic test.
- Heparin should not be started before other causes of leg swelling have been considered (Table 19.1).

Management of the swollen leg

1 Is there an infective or systemic cause of leg swelling mimicking deep-vein thrombosis (DVT)?
- Cellulitis is recognized by tenderness, erythema and induration of the skin, with fever.
- Oedema in congestive heart failure, or renal or liver disease is usually bilateral, but may initially be unilateral, or asymmetrical.

2 Is a musculoskeletal cause possible?
- Preceding trauma, or localized swelling or tenderness, or factors predisposing to Baker's cyst.
- Consider calf ultrasound or knee arthrography as first-line investigations instead of venography.
- Discuss further management with a rheumatologist or an orthopaedic surgeon.

3 Is DVT likely?
- Risk factors are present (Table 19.2); or
- evidence of pulmonary embolism (p. 155).

A heparin infusion should be started before venography (p. 386).

Treatment of proven deep-vein thrombosis

1 Bed rest with elevation of the leg for 24–48 hours.
2 Analgesia with a non-steroidal anti-inflammatory drug (NSAID) if needed.

■ **Table 19.1** Causes of leg swelling

Venous/lymphatic

- Deep-vein thrombosis
- Superficial thrombophlebitis
- IVC obstruction (e.g. by tumour)
- Varicose veins
- Postphlebitic syndrome
- Vein harvesting for coronary bypass grafting
- Congenital lymphoedema
- Dependent oedema (e.g. in paralysed limb)

Musculoskeletal

- Calf haematoma
- Ruptured Baker's cyst
- Muscle tear

Skin

- Cellulitis

Systemic

- Congestive heart failure
- Liver failure
- Renal failure
- Nephrotic syndrome
- Hypoalbuminaemia
- Chronic respiratory failure
- Pregnancy
- Idiopathic oedema of women

Drugs

- Calcium antagonists
- Drugs causing salt/water retention

IVC, Inferior vena cava.

■ **Table 19.2** Factors predisposing to deep-vein thrombosis and pulmonary embolism

- Recent surgery particularly abdominal or pelvic
- Malignant disease
- Immobility (including long car or plane journey)
- Previous DVT or pulmonary embolism
- Recent childbirth
- Severe obesity
- Use of high-oestrogen contraceptive pill
- Family history of DVT

■ **Table 19.3** Establishing the cause of deep-vein thrombosis and pulmonary embolism

- Consider risk factors (see Table 19.2)
- Check full blood count and ESR
- Women with unexplained DVT/PE should have a careful examination of the breasts, and a pelvic examination plus pelvic ultrasound
- Men should have digital examination of the prostate and measurement of prostate-specific antigen
- Patients under 40 or with a strong family history of DVT/PE should be screened for a thrombophilic disorder (deficiencies of protein C, protein S and antithrombin III; lupus anticoagulant and anticardiolipin antibodies; disorders of fibrinolysis): seek expert advice from a haematologist

ESR, Erythrocyte sedimentation rate; PE, pulmonary embolism.

3 Heparin by IV infusion (p. 386).

4 Warfarin should be started (p. 388) during heparin therapy, over-lapping for 3–4 days: during this period, check both the activated partial thromboplastin time (APTT) and International Normalized Ratio (INR) daily. Heparin can be stopped after 5 days provided the INR is > 2.0. Warfarin is usually given for 3 months after a first DVT (target INR 2.0–3.0). Indefinite treatment may be indicated after recurrent thrombo-embolism (target INR 3.0–4.5).

5 Look for the cause of the DVT (Table 19.3).

Problems

You suspected DVT but the venogram was negative

• Consider other causes of leg swelling (see Table 19.1, p. 152).

• Unexplained asymmetric leg swelling with a negative venogram is a recognized syndrome and carries a benign prognosis. No treatment is necessary.

Should every DVT be treated by anticoagulation?

• Thrombosis in the popliteal or more proximal veins of the leg should always be treated with anticoagulation (unless contraindicated).

• Whether DVT confined to the venous sinuses of the calf requires anticoagulation is controversial, particularly in the older patient.

20 Pulmonary embolism

Consider the diagnosis in any patient with unexplained:
- acute breathlessness;
- pleuritic chest pain;
- haemoptysis;
- hypotension;
- syncope.

If the patient is at risk of deep-vein thrombosis (Table 19.2, p. 153) and you cannot make a confident alternative diagnosis, treat the patient for pulmonary embolism until proven otherwise.

Priorities

1 Give oxygen and check arterial gases. Hypoxia is invariable with acute major pulmonary embolism but normal gases do not exclude a minor embolism.

2 Obtain an ECG and chest X-ray. These are principally of value in excluding alternative diagnoses (e.g. myocardial infarction, pneumonia, pneumothorax).

- The ECG will usually show only sinus tachycardia, or minor ST/T abnormalities.
- The chest X-ray may show an elevated hemidiaphragm, pulmonary oligaemia, dilatation of the pulmonary artery, a small pleural effusion or focal shadowing (the classic wedge-shaped shadow is rare).
- **A normal ECG and chest X-ray do not exclude the diagnosis.**

3 Give 5000 U of heparin by IV bolus, and start a continuous infusion (Table 60.10, p. 386).

4 If acute major embolism is suspected (systolic BP < 90 mmHg or signs of low cardiac output) follow the procedure below.

- **Connect an ECG monitor:** atrial fibrillation or flutter may occur with major pulmonary embolism and should be treated with IV digoxin (p. 20).

- **Start an infusion of colloid:** run in fluid rapidly until systolic BP is >90 mmHg. This will increase right ventricular filling and hence cardiac output.
- If the patient remains hypotensive after 500 ml of colloid has been given **start dobutamine**, at 5 µg/kg/min (p. 381) and increase it as needed up to 20 µg/kg/min until systolic BP is >90 mmHg. If systolic BP remains <90 mmHg, noradrenaline should be given (p. 374).
- **Decide whether thrombolytic therapy should be given (Tables 20.1 and 20.2).** Most deaths from acute major pulmonary embolism occur within 1 hour, so pulmonary angiography is rarely practicable. Echocardiography is helpful if it can be done immediately.

Further management

1 Continue heparin by infusion (see Table 60.10, p. 386). Check the activated partial thromboplastin time (APTT) at 6 hours and adjust the dose as required, aiming for an APTT 1.5–2.5 × control.

2 Confirm the diagnosis. Further investigation to confirm or exclude pulmonary embolism is essential. A scheme for this is shown in Fig. 20.2.

3 Warfarin should be started (see Table 60.13, p. 388) during heparin therapy, overlapping for 3–4 days: during this period, check both the APTT and International Normalized Ratio (INR) daily. Heparin can be stopped after 5 days provided the INR is >2.0. Warfarin is usually given for 3 months after a first pulmonary embolism (target INR

■ **Table 20.1** Thrombolytic therapy for acute major pulmonary embolism: criteria to be met

- Systolic BP <90 mmHg after standard treatment for 30–60 min
- Clinically definite embolism (compatible clinical picture, risk factor(s) for thrombo-embolism present (Table 19.2, p. 153), no other diagnosis likely)
- No contraindication to thrombolytic therapy (Table 12.4, p. 110)

■ **Table 20.2** Thrombolytic therapy for acute major pulmonary embolism:
regimens

Thrombolytic therapy can be given via a peripheral or central vein. If
pulmonary angiography has been performed, leave the angiography catheter
in place because of the risk of bleeding from the puncture site

Standard regimens

Streptokinase
- Loading dose: 600 000 U IV over 30 min
- Maintenance dose: 100 000 U/hour IV for 24 hours

Urokinase
- Loading dose: 4 400 U/kg IV over 10 minutes
- Maintenance dose: 4 400 U/kg/hour IV for 12 hours

Check the TT or APTT 3–4 hours after stopping streptokinase or urokinase.
When TT/APTT are less than twice control, restart the heparin infusion

Experimental regimen

Alteplase
- 100 mg IV over 2 hours*

TT, Thrombin time; APTT, activated partial thromboplastin time.
* Goldhaber SZ *et al. Lancet* 1988; 2: 293–8.

2.0–3.0). Indefinite treatment may be indicated after recurrent
thromboembolism (target INR 3.0–4.5).
4 Look for a cause for the pulmonary embolism (see Table 19.3,
p. 153).

a Acute major

- sudden circulatory collapse
- central chest pain
- hyperventilation
- engorged neck veins
- ECG: sometimes RV strain pattern
- CXR: usually unhelpful
- Angio: shows obstruction
- Scan: not done

b Acute minor

With infarction:

- pleuritic pain
- haemoptysis
- effusion
- fever
- hyperventilation
- CXR: segmental collapse/
  consolidation

Without infarction:

- may be silent
- dyspnoea
- fever
- ECG: unhelpful
- Angio: usually shows obstruction
- Scan: usually reflects obstruction

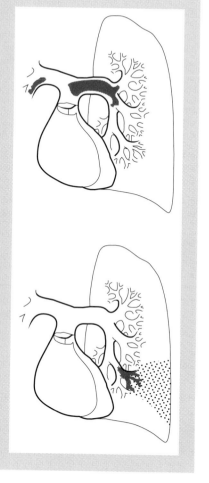

Fig. 20.1 Acute major vs acute minor pulmonary embolism. From Brewis RAL. *Lecture Notes on Respiratory Disease.* 3rd edn. Oxford: Blackwell Scientific Publications, 1985.

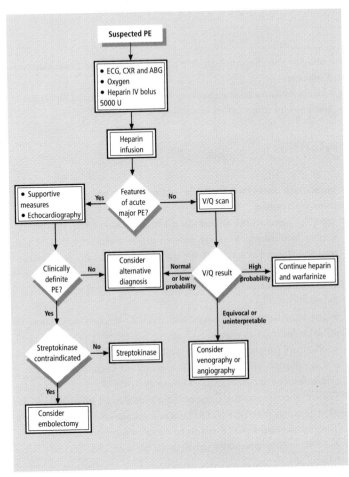

Fig. 20.2 Investigation and management of suspected pulmonary embolism.

21 Acute asthma

- Consider the diagnosis in any patient with **acute breathlessness and wheeze**.
- Always measure peak expiratory flow rate and arterial blood gases.
- The severity of an attack is easily underestimated.

Priorities

1 **Immediate assessment of the patient with an exacerbation of asthma is essential.**
2 **Look for signs of life threatening asthma (Table 21.1). If present:**
   - give salbutamol 5 mg by oxygen-driven nebulizer — make sure that the flow rate is correct for the nebulizer (usually 6–8 l/min);
   - give hydrocortisone 200 mg IV;
   - call an anaesthetist in case urgent intubation and ventilation are needed;
   - check arterial blood gases and monitor oxygen saturation by pulse oximetry if available;
   - continue treatment as below; some patients will improve rapidly but ventilation will be needed if the patient becomes increasingly exhausted or Pa_{CO_2} remains > 7 kPa or $Pa_{O_2} < 7$ kPa on 60% oxygen.
3 For other patients, the decision to admit should be based on the peak expiratory flow rate (PEFR) (as a percentage of predicted (p. 393) or best known) and the response to nebulized bronchodilator.
   - **PEFR $>75\%$ predicted:** give usual inhaler and if stable after 60 min, discharge.
   - **PEFR $>50\%$ but $<75\%$ predicted:** give salbutamol 5 mg by oxygen-driven nebulizer. Reassess at 30 min. If PEFR is now $>75\%$, discharge. If not, repeat nebulizer and give prednisolone 40 mg PO. Reassess at 60 min. Admit if PEFR is not $>60\%$ and the patient is not improving.
   - **PEFR $<50\%$ predicted or best known: admit. (a)** Give oxygen (8–10 l/min by MC mask or equivalent) and nebulized salbutamol

■ **Table 21.1** Acute asthma: clinical features

Life-threatening attack

- Silent chest, feeble respiratory effort
- Bradycardia or hypotension
- Exhaustion, confusion or coma

Severe attack

- Unable to speak in full sentences
- Respiratory rate > 25/min
- Pulse rate > 120/min
- Pulsus paradoxus (p. 149) > 20 mmHg (not always found)

■ **Table 21.2** Arterial blood gases in acute asthma

Severity of asthma	Pao_2*	$Paco_2$	pH
Mild	> 10	< 4	> 7.45
Moderate	8–10	< 4	> 7.45
Severe	< 8	4.5–6	7.35–7.45
Exhaustion	< 7	> 6	< 7.35

* Pao_2 must be related to the inspired oxygen concentration. The values given are with the patient breathing air.

(5 mg nebule). If nebules are not available, dilute to a total volume of 3 ml using normal saline – do not use water as a diluent; **(b)** give hydrocortisone 200 mg IV; **(c)** recheck PEFR after 15 min; **(d)** measure arterial blood gases (Table 21.2) and arrange a chest X-ray; **(e)** repeat nebulized salbutamol if no improvement; **(f)** If life-threatening signs develop, call an anaesthetist and arrange transfer to the intensive-therapy unit; put in an arterial line as frequent blood gas sampling may be required.

Further management

1 **Confirm the diagnosis by:**
- positive features in the history (Table 21.3);

■ **Table 21.3** Features supporting a diagnosis of asthma

- Previous similar episodes of breathlessness or wheeze responding to bronchodilator therapy
- Diurnal (particularly with nocturnal symptoms) and/or seasonal variation in symptoms
- Wheeze provoked by exercise or allergen exposure
- Eczema or hayfever
- Family history of asthma
- 'Chestiness' or 'wheezy bronchitis' in childhood

■ **Table 21.4** Causes of acute breathlessness and wheeze

- Acute asthma
- Acute infective exacerbation of chronic airflow limitation (p. 166)
- Pulmonary oedema (p. 136)
- Pulmonary embolism (p. 155)
- Anaphylactic reaction (p. 296)
- Upper airways obstruction (see Table 21.5)

- the exclusion of other causes of breathlessness and wheeze (Table 21.4). Upper airways obstruction (Table 21.5) should always be considered in patients with no history of previous similar attacks. If you suspect this, seek expert advice from an ENT surgeon or chest physician.

2 Steroid therapy. Bronchial inflammation and oedema are important factors in acute asthma.

- Give hydrocortisone 200 mg IV stat in moderate or severe attacks.
- At the same time start oral prednisolone 40 mg daily.
- Start inhaled steroid before discharge (e.g. Becloforte, 2 puffs morning and night) and check inhaler technique.
- Stop prednisolone after 10–14 days (taper if the patient has previously been receiving oral steroid).

3 Oxygen.

- Start with 60% humidified oxygen via a controlled delivery mask.
- Increase if necessary to achieve Pa_{O_2} >10 kPa (75 mmHg).

■ **Table 21.5** Upper airways obstruction in adults

Causes

- Inhalation of foreign body
- Tumours of larynx and trachea (preceding hoarseness)
- Angioedema (associated urticaria)
- Acute epiglottitis

Clues to the diagnosis

- Stridor (inspiratory wheeze)
- No response to bronchodilator
- Raised Pa_{CO_2}

4 Bronchodilator therapy.

- Give nebulized salbutamol 2.5–5 mg (nebule or 0.5–1 ml of nebulizer solution diluted to 3 ml in normal saline) 4-hourly.
- If the response is poor, add ipratropium 250–500 µg (nebule or 1–2 ml of nebulizer solution) 4-hourly. The two can be given together, or alternately every 2 hours.
- If the response remains poor, an IV infusion should be started. If the patient is not taking an oral theophylline preparation, give aminophylline (Table 21.6): monitor plasma levels if possible. If the patient is already taking theophylline, give salbutamol (Table 21.6).

Other points

Monitoring progress

Peak expiratory flow rate should be measured initially 4-hourly (before and after bronchodilator therapy). **Arterial gases** should be rechecked:

- if Pa_{CO_2} was above 5 kPa on admission (recheck 20–30 min after institution of treatment);
- if the PEFR is not improving;
- if the patient's clinical condition worsens.

■ **Table 21.6** Bronchodilator infusions in acute severe asthma

Aminophylline

Loading dose: 250–500 mg (5 mg/kg) IV over 10–15 min. Ensure the patient is on supplemental oxygen to reduce the risk of arrhythmia

Maintenance dose: 0.5 mg/kg/hour by IV infusion. If you cannot check levels, halve the dose in patients with congestive heart failure or liver disease. **For an average sized adult, add 250 mg to 1 l of saline or dextrose 5% and infuse over 8 hours**

The **therapeutic range** for theophylline is 10–20 mg/l. **Nausea and vomiting** are common toxic effects

Salbutamol

Add 5 mg (5 ml of 1 mg/ml solution) to 500 ml normal saline or 5% dextrose (giving a salbutamol concentration of 10 µg/ml)

Start at 1 ml/min, increasing up to 3 ml/min if necessary

Monitor plasma potassium: hypokalaemia may occur

Antibiotics

Only a minority of asthma attacks are provoked by infection, and most of these by viral infections. Antibiotics are not routinely required.

• Give where there is good evidence of respiratory infection – fever, purulent (green) sputum or focal shadowing on the chest X-ray. Yellow/green sputum may be due to eosinophils and a raised white cell count to steroids.

• The choice of antibiotics is as for pneumonia (see Table 23.4, p. 176).

Physiotherapy

Physiotherapy should not be given routinely.

Plasma potassium

Salbutamol and steroids may result in significant hypokalaemia. Check electrolytes the day after admission and give potassium supplements if potassium is < 3.5 mmol/l.

Fluids

Patients are frequently dehydrated on admission. Ensure a fluid intake of 2–3 l/day, given IV if necessary.

Failure to improve

Consider the following possibilities.

1 Wrong diagnosis: other causes of acute breathlessness and wheeze are given in Table 21.4.

2 Untreated bacterial infection.

3 Pneumothorax.

4 Inadequate therapy.

- Check that the nebulizer is set up correctly – it should nebulize 3 ml in 10–15 min. Most are run at 6–8 l/min: at lower rates the droplets are too big to be inhaled adequately.
- Nebulized salbutamol can be given 2-hourly if necessary.
- Nebulized ipratropium can be added.

22 Acute exacerbation of chronic airflow limitation

Consider the diagnosis in any patient with **chronic airflow limitation** who develops **increased breathlessness, confusion or drowsiness**.

Priorities

1 Your clinical assessment (including usual functional capacity of the patient, Table 22.1) is directed at establishing **whether symptoms are due to an infective exacerbation or another cause** (Table 22.2).

- The working diagnosis of **infective exacerbation** is based on an **increase in sputum volume** or the development of **purulent sputum**.

2 Check peak expiratory flow rate. Give salbutamol 5.0 mg and ipratropium 500 μg by air-driven nebulizer.

3 Check arterial blood gases and pH. If respiratory failure is present ($Pao_2 < 8$ kPa) give oxygen (initially 28% by Ventimask or 2 l/min by nasal cannulae). Other investigations required urgently are given in Table 22.3.

4 Any pneumothorax unless very small must be drained (p. 348).

Further management of infective exacerbation

This consists of bronchodilator therapy, oxygen, antibiotics and steroids (in some cases). Physiotherapy is of little value unless sputum is copious: otherwise it increases hypoxia and does not speed recovery.

Bronchodilator therapy

- **Salbutamol** 2.5–5 mg (nebule or 0.5–1 ml of nebulizer solution diluted to 3 ml in normal saline) 4-hourly, plus:

■ **Table 22.1** Functional assessment in chronic airflow limitation

- Distance walked on the flat
- How many stairs without stopping?
- How many pillows at night?
- Usual volume of sputum produced
- Frequency of acute exacerbations
- Ever ventilated?
- Previous lung-function tests (from the notes)
- Concurrent illness especially cardiac disease

■ **Table 22.2** Chronic airflow limitation: causes of increased dyspnoea

- Infective, exacerbation
- Pneumonia (focal shadowing on chest X-ray; see p. 173)
- Pneumothorax (differentiate from bulla; see p. 179)
- Pulmonary embolism (suspect if there is pleuritic chest pain with clear lung fields; see p. 155)
- Sedative drugs
- Mucus plugging with segmental or lobar collapse
- Cardiac disease (e.g. myocardial infarction, arrythmia)

■ **Table 22.3** Urgent investigation in acute exacerbation of chronic airflow limitation

- Chest X-ray
- Arterial blood gases and pH
- ECG
- Peak expiratory flow rate (see p. 393 for normal values)
- Sputum culture
- Blood culture if febrile or focal shadowing on chest X-ray
- Urea, sodium and potassium
- Full blood count

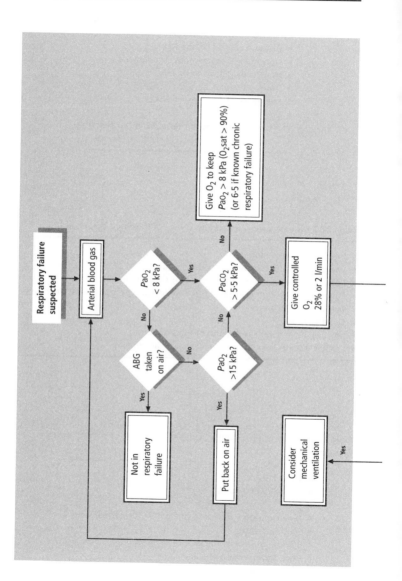

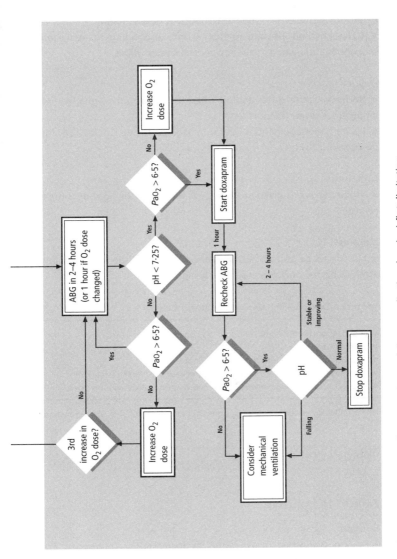

Fig. 22.1 Management of acute respiratory failure complicating chronic airflow limitation.

• **Ipratropium** 250–500 µg (nebule or 1–2 ml of nebulizer solution) by air-driven nebuliser 4-hourly (2-hourly if needed) and:
• **Aminophylline infusion** (p. 164) if not responding to nebulized bronchodilators and not already on oral theophylline.

Oxygen

• **Recheck arterial gases and pH** 1 hour after starting oxygen (earlier if conscious level deteriorates).
• Further management is given in Fig. 22.1. See Table 22.4 for doxapram infusion.

Antibiotics

• Initial therapy is given in Table 22.5. Modify in the light of culture results.

Steroids

If known to be steroid responsive, or showing little improvement after 48 hours, start prednisolone 40 mg daily PO.

■ **Table 22.4** Doxapram infusion in respiratory failure

• A 500 ml bottle contains 2 mg/ml in 5% dextrose
• Start infusion at 1 ml/min
• Recheck arterial gases and pH after 1 hour
• If respiratory rate is < 20 breaths/min, increase infusion to 2 ml/min
• Recheck arterial gases and pH 2- to 4-hourly until improvement is established

---

NB: usually causes some degree of agitation. May interact with aminophylline.

Problems

Failure to improve

Consider:

• **wrong diagnosis:** other causes of increased breathlessness are given in Table 22.2;

■ **Table 22.5** Initial antibiotic therapy for infective exacerbation of chronic airflow limitation

---

- **Amoxycillin** 500 mg 8-hourly PO; **or**
- **Trimethoprim** 200 mg 12-hourly PO; **or**
- **Ciprofloxacin** 500 mg 12-hourly PO

- **untreated bacterial infection;**
- **sputum retention:** acetylcysteine (20% w/v 2–5 ml 6-hourly by nebulizer) may loosen mucus plugs;
- **pneumothorax;**
- **inadequate therapy:** nebulized salbutamol and ipratropium can be given 2-hourly if necessary, or salbutamol can be given by IV infusion (see Table 21.6, p. 164).

Respiratory failure unresponsive to oxygen and doxapram

Mechanical ventilation may be indicated but should be discussed with a chest physician and an anaesthetist. It is contraindicated by poor basal functional capacity (see Table 22.1, p. 167) and carries the risk of pneumothorax induced by barotrauma and of ventilator dependence.

Arrhythmias

- Check plasma potassium: salbutamol and steroids may result in significant hypokalaemia. Give potassium supplements if potassium is < 3.5 mmol/l.
- Treat atrial fibrillation/flutter with amiodarone or digoxin (see Table 2.10, p. 20).
- For multifocal atrial tachycardia (p. 22) consider verapamil if the ventricular rate is consistently > 110/min. DC cardioversion is ineffective.

Congestive heart failure

• Is usually due to pulmonary heart disease and will improve as respiratory function improves. If in doubt, arrange echocardiography to exclude left-sided heart disease.

• Treat with diuretic, avoiding overdiuresis.

23 Pneumonia

Consider pneumonia in any patient with:
- **acute dyspnoea and fever;**
- **signs of sepsis;**
- **acute confusional state.**

Factors predisposing to pneumonia are given in Table 23.1. Examination may be normal (listen over the lung apices and laterally) and a chest X-ray should always be obtained.

Priorities

1 Check arterial blood gases and give oxygen if needed.
- In the absence of hypoxia, look at the $Paco_2$: a low $Paco_2$ indicates the need for oxygen in a patient working hard to maintain a normal Pao_2.

2 Check the BP: if systolic BP is < 90 mmHg, put in a peripheral line and give a fluid challenge of 250 ml of colloid over 15 min. If the BP does not increase, put in a central line. See p. 34 for further management of hypotension.

3 Investigation of the patient with suspected pneumonia is given in Table 23.2.
- Features associated with an increased risk of death are given in Table 23.3.

4 Start antibiotic therapy as soon as blood has been taken for culture.
- Your initial choice of antibiotic depends on the clinical setting (Table 23.4).
- Antibiotics can be given orally unless there is vomiting, fever $> 38°C$ or significant hypoxia ($Pao_2 < 8$ kPa) when they should be given IV.

5 Transfer the patient to the intensive-therapy unit (ITU) if:
- respiratory rate > 30 min or patient exhausted;
- $Pao_2 < 8$ kPa (60 mmHg) despite 60% oxygen;

■ **Table 23.1** Factors predisposing to pneumonia

- Chronic airways disease (chronic bronchitis, bronchiectasis)
- Bronchial obstruction due to carcinoma or inhaled foreign body
- Chronic alcoholism
- Immunocompromised

Inhalation pneumonia

- Recent anaesthetic
- Cardiopulmonary resuscitation
- Diabetic ketoacidosis
- Alcohol intoxication
- Impaired gag/cough reflex, e.g. due to stroke

■ **Table 23.2** Urgent investigation in suspected pneumonia

- Chest X-ray*
- Arterial blood gases and pH
- Full blood count
- Blood culture (positive in 80% of pneumococcal pneumonias)
- Urea, sodium and potassium
- Sputum for Gram stain and culture
- Pleural fluid (if present) for Gram stain and culture

* The distribution of shadowing on the chest X-ray is a poor guide to the causative organism. Other features to look for are; **(a) pleural effusion** – if present, aspirate a sample and send for Gram stain and culture; **(b) cavitation** – particularly associated with tuberculosis and *Staphylococcus aureus* infection, but also may occur with Gram negative and anaerobic infections; **(c) pneumothorax** – may occur in cavitating pneumonias and is particularly associated with *Pneumocystis carinii* pneumonia (p. 284).

- $Pa_{CO_2} > 6\,kPa$ (45 mmHg);
- Systolic BP < 90 mmHg despite IV fluids.

Put in an arterial line, central venous line and urinary catheter. Discuss the need for mechanical ventilation with an ITU physician or anaesthetist.

■ **Table 23.3** Clinical and laboratory features associated with an increased risk of death from pneumonia

Clinical	Laboratory
Respiratory rate > 30/min	Blood urea > 7 mmol/l
Diastolic BP < 60 mmHg	Albumin < 35 g/l
Age > 60 years	PaO_2 < 8 kPa (60 mmHg)
Underlying disease	WBC > 20 or < 4×10^9/l
Confusion	Bacteraemia
Atrial fibrillation	
Multilobar involvement	

WBC, White blood cell count.

Reference:
British Thoracic Society. Community-acquired pneumonia in adults in British hospitals in 1982–1983: a survey of aetiology, mortality, prognostic factors and outcome. *Quart J Med* 1987; 62: 195–220.

Further management

Supportive treatment consists of:

1 Oxygen: should be given humidified and continued until Pao_2 is > 8 kPa (60 mmHg) with the patient breathing air, or oxygen saturation is > 90%.

2 Fluid balance: insensible losses are greater than normal due to fever (500 ml/day/°C) and tachypnoea. Patients with severe pneumonia should receive IV fluids (2–3 l/day) with a daily check of urea and electrolytes if abnormal on admission. Monitor the central venous pressure (CVP) if the patient is oliguric or if plasma urea is > 15 mmol/l.

3 Analgesia for pleuritic pain: give paracetamol or a non-steroidal anti-inflammatory drug (NSAID) such as indomethacin.

4 Physiotherapy: if patients are producing sputum, but having trouble expectorating it. Patients with bronchiectasis should have physiotherapy started on admission.

5 Bronchodilator therapy with salbutamol (p. 164) if there is wheeze.

■ **Table 23.4** Initial 'blind' antibiotic therapy for pneumonia

Mild community-acquired pneumonia

- Amoxycillin 500 mg 8-hourly PO; or
- Erythromycin 500 mg 6-hourly PO if penicillin allergy, previous poor response to amoxycillin or features to suggest 'atypical' pneumonia (Appendix 1)

Severe community-acquired pneumonia

- Amoxycillin 500 mg 8-hourly IV; plus
- Erythromycin 500 mg 6-hourly IV (best given by a long line or central line to avoid thrombophlebitis); plus
- Flucloxacillin 500 mg 6-hourly IV if staphylococcal pneumonia is a possibility: (a) if there is recent influenza; (b) cavitation on the chest X-ray (but consider the possibility of TB); (c) Gram stain of sputum shows clusters of Gram-positive cocci

Severe hospital-acquired pneumonia

- Third generation cephalosporin; or
- Aminoglycoside plus antipseudomonal penicillin (e.g. gentamicin plus azlocillin) if *Pseudomonas* infection possible (neutropenic, bronchiectasis, mechanical ventilation)

Inhalation pneumonia

- Benzyl penicillin plus metronidazole if community-acquired
- Third generation cephalosporin if hospital-acquired

Nebulized normal saline may be helpful when sputum is thick and difficult to expectorate.

Problems

The patient is no better despite 48 hours of antibiotic therapy

- **Repeat the chest X-ray** — are there any new findings such as cavitation or pleural effusion? If pleural fluid is now present, this should be aspirated and sent for Gram stain and culture. If the fluid is at all cloudy, drain completely and treat as empyema: seek expert advice from a chest physician.

- **Consider pulmonary tuberculosis:** send sputum for Ziehl−Nielson stain. If no sputum is being produced, consider fibreoptic bronchoscopy. A Mantoux skin test (0.1 ml or 1 in 10 000 intradermally) may be performed, but interpretation can be difficult − a strongly positive test is good evidence of active infection, but a negative reaction can occur in the presence of active infection.
- **Consider the possibility of immunocompromise** or HIV/AIDS related pneumonia (p. 284).
- **Consider non-infective causes of chest X-ray shadowing** such as pulmonary infarction, pulmonary oedema or bronchial carcinoma.
- **Seek expert advice from a chest physician** regarding fibreoptic bronchoscopy (Table 23.5) and further management.

The postoperative patient − pneumonia or pulmonary embolism?

Acute dyspnoea and fever are features of both. Pneumonia is favoured by:

- initial fever $> 39°C$;

■ **Table 23.5** Indications for fibreoptic bronchoscopy in the patient with pneumonia

Early bronchoscopy

- Suspected foreign-body inhalation
- No organism identified from blood or sputum and patient not responding to antibiotics
- Cavitating pneumonia with negative sputum microscopy and culture
- Lobar or segmental collapse with significant hypoxia

Late bronchoscopy

- Persistent (> 1 week) segmental or lobar collapse
- Slow resolution of symptoms and signs (NB: chest X-ray shadowing may take up to 6 weeks to clear completely)
- Recurrent pneumonia in the same site

- white cell count $> 15 \times 10^9/l$;
- purulent sputum.

If you remain uncertain, treat for both conditions until a ventilation/perfusion scan can be performed. See p. 155 for further management of pulmonary embolism.

Appendix 1

■ **Table 23.6** Typical features of pneumococcal, mycoplasmal and *Legionella* pneumonias

Feature	Pneumococcal	Mycoplasmal	Legionella
Onset	Acute	Subacute	Subacute
Initial symptoms	Rigor	Cough Sore throat	Cough Headache
Temperature (°C)	39–40	<39	39–40
Chest signs	Bronchial breathing common Pleural rub common	Focal crackles common Bronchial breathing uncommon Radiological involvement greater than signs	
WBC ($\times 10^9/l$)	>15	<15	<15
Differential WBC count	Neutrophilia	Normal	Neutrophilia
Useful clues	Herpes labialis	Young adult Neurological symptoms Epidemic	Hyponatraemia Confusion Gastrointestinal symptoms Travel abroad Epidemic

WBC, White cell count.

24 Pneumothorax

Consider the diagnosis in any patient with:
- **sudden breathlessness or chest pain**, particularly in young, otherwise-fit adults and following invasive procedures, e.g. subclavian vein puncture, lung biopsy, chest aspiration;
- **acute exacerbations of asthma or chronic airways obstruction** – pneumothorax may be painless and contribute to respiratory failure;
- **hypoxia or an increase in inflation pressure if mechanically ventilated** – asymmetry of chest expansion is a useful clue.

Priorities

If the patient has signs of a pneumothorax and is hypotensive (systolic BP < 90 mmHg), suspect a tension pneumothorax.
- Insert the largest cannula to hand into the second intercostal space in the midclavicular line on the side with absent or reduced breath sounds: if air rushes out, leave the cannula in place until a chest drain is inserted.
- Insert an intercostal drain immediately.

Further management

1 **Obtain a chest X-ray.** You may rupture the lung if you mistake an emphysematous bulla for a small pneumothorax. Points in favour of a bulla are:
- adhesions between the lung and the parietal pleura;
- a scallop-shaped edge to the cavity;
- faint markings over the lucency caused by the lung enfolding the bulla;
- the presence of other bullae.

If you suspected a pneumothorax, but the chest X-ray appears normal, see Table 24.1.

■ **Table 24.1** Apparently normal chest X-ray in suspected pneumothorax

If there is no obvious lung margin, recheck:

- The lung apices
- The right border of the heart

In the supine patient look for:

- Unusually sharp appearance of the cardiac border or diaphragm with increased transradiancy of the adjacent parts of the thorax and abdomen
- A vertical line parallel to the chest wall (caused by retraction of the middle lobe from the chest wall)
- A diagonal line from the heart to the costophrenic angle

2 Check arterial blood gases in severely dyspnoeic patients and those with chronic lung disease.

3 Management options (Fig. 24.1). If the pneumothorax is left alone or managed by needle aspiration:

- Advise the patient to return immediately in the event of deterioration and to avoid air travel until the chest X-ray is normal;
- Arrange a further chest X-ray in 7–10 days.

4 Surgical advice should be sought if:

- there are bilateral pneumothoraces;
- the lung fails to re-expand on intercostal tube drainage;
- there is a history of two or more previous pneumothoraces on the same side as the current episode;
- there is a history of pneumothorax on the other side.

Appendix 1: needle aspiration of a small pneumothorax

1 Identify the third–fourth intercostal space in the midaxillary line.
2 Infiltrate with lignocaine down to and around the pleura over the pneumothorax.
3 Connect a 21G (green) needle to a three-way tap and a 60 ml syringe.

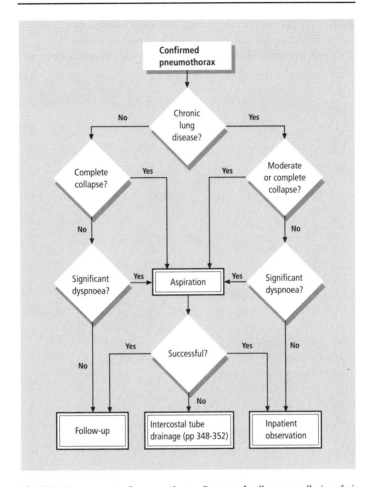

Fig. 24.1 Management of pneumothorax. Degree of collapse: small, rim of air around lung; moderate, lung collapsed halfway towards heart border; complete, airless lung, separate from diaphragm. **Needle aspiration, see p. 180; intercostal tube drainage, see p. 348.** From Miller AC, Harvey JE. Guidelines for the management of spontaneous pneumothorax. *BMJ* 1993; 307: 114–16.

4 With the patient semirecumbent, insert the needle into the pleural space. Withdraw air and expel it via the three-way tap.

5 Obtain a chest X-ray to confirm resolution of the pneumothorax.

25 Haemoptysis

- Every patient presenting with haemoptysis should have the cause established (Table 25.1). If the diagnosis is not clear, refer to a chest physician for further investigation.
- When there is doubt from the history, haemoptysis can be distinguished from haematemesis by its colour and pH (haemoptysis is bright red and alkaline; haematemesis is brown and acid). Bleeding from the nasopharynx may also be confused with haemoptysis: if this is possible, ask the opinion of an ENT surgeon.

Priorities

Patients with massive haemoptysis (> 1000 ml in 24 hours)

There is a risk of death from exsanguination or drowning.

1 Call an anaesthetist: endotracheal intubation may be needed to allow suctioning of the airway and adequate ventilation.

2 Put in a large-bore venous cannula and take blood for urgent cross-match and other investigations (Table 25.2).

3 Start an infusion of colloid until blood is available.

4 Contact a thoracic surgeon for advice on further management. Bleeding may occasionally be stopped through a rigid bronchoscope, but usually requires resection of the bleeding segment or lobe.

Other patients

1 Investigation is given in Table 25.2. Further management is directed by the likely diagnosis.

2 It may not be necessary to admit the patient if the diagnosis is clear and the patient stable (e.g. bronchial carcinoma, bronchiectasis). Seek expert advice from a chest physician if you are in doubt. If you discharge the patient, arrange early follow-up.

■ **Table 25.1** Causes of haemoptysis

Cause	Comment
Bronchial carcinoma	Persistent blood-streaking of mucoid sputum; weight loss
Tuberculosis	Blood-streaking of purulent sputum; weight loss; fever
Bronchiectasis	Blood-streaking of copious purulent sputum; chronic sputum production; previous episodes of haemoptysis occurring over months or years
Acute bronchitis	Blood-streaking of mucopurulent sputum
Pneumonia (p. 173)	'Rusty' sputum; acute illness with fever and breathlessness, signs of consolidation
Lung abscess	Blood-streaking of purulent sputum; fever; pleuritic chest pain
Pulmonary infarction (p. 155)	Gross blood not mixed with sputum; pleuritic chest pain and breathlessness; at risk of deep-vein thrombosis (see Table 19.2, p. 153)
Pulmonary oedema (p. 136)	Frothy blood-tinged sputum; severe breathlessness; associated cardiac disease
Lung contusion	Preceding chest trauma
Mycetoma	Fungal ball on chest X-ray; previous pulmonary tuberculosis
Vascular malformation	Recurrent haemoptysis; Osler–Weber–Rendu syndrome with multiple telangiectasia
Bronchial adenoma	Recurrent haemoptysis; otherwise-well woman
Bleeding tendency	Haemoptysis resulting from persistent coughing; bleeding from other sites
Pulmonary vasculitis	Wegener's granulomatosis; Goodpasture syndrome
Pulmonary hypertension	Mitral stenosis; primary pulmonary hypertension; Eisenmenger syndrome

■ **Table 25.2** Investigation of the patient with haemoptysis

Massive haemoptysis

- Full blood count
- Clotting screen
- Urgent cross-match 4 units
- Urea, sodium and potassium
- Arterial blood gases
- Chest X-ray when stable

Other patients

- Chest X-ray
- Arterial blood gases (if pleuritic chest pain or breathlessness)
- Sputum for Gram and Ziehl–Nielson stain, culture and cytology
- Full blood count
- ESR
- Clotting screen if bleeding tendency suspected
- Urea, sodium and potassium
- Urinalysis
- ECG (if pulmonary oedema suspected)

Further investigation

- Bronchoscopy
- Computed tomography of thorax

ESR, Erythrocyte sedimentation rate.

26 Hyperventilation

• Hyperventilation (Pa_{CO_2} < 4.3 kPa (32 mmHg)) is a respiratory response to organic lung disease, hypoxia, sepsis, metabolic acidosis, acute central nervous system disorders, or pain.

• In patients without significant organic disease (primary hyperventilation) it may present acutely with panic and carpopedal spasm, or with recurrent breathlessness, chest pain or dizziness.

• It is vital to exclude an underlying organic cause of tachypnoea before treating as primary hyperventilation: investigations required are given in Table 26.1.

Panic and carpopedal spasm

1 Take the pulse and BP and listen to the chest. Check the oxygen saturation by pulse oximetery (if less than 95%, consider organic disease).

2 If the patient is unable to control their breathing, place a paper bag lightly over the mouth to induce carbon dioxide re-breathing. (If applied too firmly it may exacerbate the panic and hyperventilation.)

3 If this fails, give diazepam (Diazemuls) in 2 mg aliquots IV until sedation occurs. If this is required, the arterial blood gases must first be checked to exclude a respiratory cause for hyperventilation and the patient must either be admitted or accompanied home (after observation).

Hyperventilation as the cause of recurrent symptoms

1 Suspect in the patient with an irregular, thoracic, sighing respiratory pattern. Symptoms which point strongly to the diagnosis (and which may not be volunteered) are given in Table 26.2.

■ **Table 26.1** Investigation in suspected hyperventilation

- **Chest X-ray** (check for a small pneumothorax, signs of infection, or hyperinflated lungs)
- **ECG** (hyperventilation may induce T wave changes and even ST depression, but ischaemic heart disease must be excluded first if these abnormalities are present)
- **Arterial blood gases and pH** (see p. 398 for interpretation)
- **Peak expiratory flow rate** (airflow limitation is a common cause of hyperventilation (see p. 393 for normal values)
- **Blood glucose** (if > 10 mmol/l, always consider diabetic ketoacidosis, p. 253)
- **Urea, sodium and potassium**
- **Full blood count**

■ **Table 26.2** Symptoms which may be associated with hyperventilation in the absence of organic disease

Breathlessness

- At rest especially sitting, after bending or immediately after lying down
- With trivial exertion, e.g. one or two steps, or 50 m on the flat
- Talking or eating
- Situational, e.g. in confined spaces
- With emotion
- Feeling of having to take gulps of air
- Associated sighing or throat clearing

Chest pain

- At rest or after exertion
- Relieved by exertion
- Left submammary or axillary
- Continuous ache or jabs
- Variable character, site and duration
- Duration > 20 min

Others

- Fatigue
- Digital or circumoral paraesthaesiae
- Dizziness; occasionally syncope
- Anxiety
- Poor sleep

■ **Table 26.3** Hyperventilation provocation test

- Ask the patient to take deep breaths at 30–40 breaths/min for up to 2 min.
- Ask which symptoms were reproduced; was the sensation similar or an exact reproduction?
- The test is positive if the index symptoms are reproduced exactly

■ **Table 26.4** Breathing exercises in the treatment of hyperventilation

- Place one hand on the chest and the other on the abdomen
- Recognize diaphragmatic breathing when the top hand remains still and the lower hand moves out during inspiration
- Breathe slowly (8–10 breaths/min) to a regular ryhthm – slowly in – 2,3 – slowly out – 2,3 – etc.
- Resist taking gasps

2 Exclude organic disease clinically and by investigations (see Table 26.1).

3 Perform a hyperventilation provocation test (Table 26.3).

4 Treatment consists of:

- reassurance and explanation, which are often sufficient to defuse an alarming symptom: a positive provocation test is useful in demonstrating the underlying mechanism:
- simple breathing exercises (Table 26.4), or referral to a specialist physiotherapist if these fail.
- addressing any underlying psychological precipitants.

27 Stroke

- The working diagnosis of stroke is based on the **sudden or rapid onset of a focal neurological deficit**.
- Completed stroke is arbitrarily distinguished from transient ischaemic attack (Chapter 28) by the persistence of symptoms for > 24 hours.

Priorities

1 If the patient is unconscious, initial resuscitation is as for coma from any cause (p. 53). Coma at onset usually indicates cerebral haemorrhage.

2 Your clinical assessment (Table 27.1) and investigations (Table 27.2) are directed at answering the following four questions.

- **Is this a stroke** – and not some other illness that may mimic stroke (Table 27.3)?
- **Where is the stroke** (Table 27.4)?
- **Is the stroke due to haemorrhage or infarction?** Around 80% of strokes are due to infarction. Headache, vomiting and coma at onset are more common in haemorrhagic stroke, but **accurate differentiation requires computed tomography (CT)**.
- **Does the stroke have a potentially treatable cause** (Table 27.5)?

Further management

1 Specific therapy to increase cerebral perfusion or protect the brain from ischaemic injury.

- Many therapies have been tried (e.g. corticosteroids, glycerol, naftidrofuryl, calcium antagonists, haemodilution) but none have as yet been shown to improve outcome in large randomized trials.
- Thrombolytic agents, heparin and aspirin are currently being tested (International Stroke Trial, started 1993).

■ **Table 27.1** Key points in the clinical assessment of stroke

Point	Comment
Onset of symptoms	Progression over days or weeks suggests mass lesion
Headache or vomiting at onset	Suggests cerebral haemorrhage
Preceding TIA or amaurosis fugax	Suggests cerebral infarction
Fever at presentation	Consider brain abscess, meningitis (p. 204), encephalitis (p. 210), endocarditis, and cerebral malaria in patients at risk (p. 307)
Reduced conscious level	More common in cerebral haemorrhage, but may occur in cerebral infarction with brain swelling
Neck stiffness	May occur in cerebral haemorrhage, but consider meningitis (p. 204) and subarachnoid haemorrhage (p. 200)

■ **Table 27.2** Urgent investigation of the patient with stroke

Blood glucose
Full blood count
Sickle solubility test if appropriate (p. 299)
Urea, sodium and potassium
Blood culture if febrile or endocarditis suspected
ECG (? atrial fibrillation, LV hypertrophy, myocardial infarction)
Chest X-ray (? lung neoplasm, cardiac enlargement)
CT scan on admission:
• **If there is doubt about the diagnosis of stroke;** no history available; gradual onset; or progressive symptoms
• **If there may be an intracranial haematoma or obstructive hydrocephalus needing surgical intervention;** suspected subarachnoid haemorrhage (p. 200); suspected chronic subdural haematoma; suspected cerebellar stroke; associated head injury; or patient on warfarin or with bleeding tendency

LV, Left ventricle; CT, computed tomography.

■ **Table 27.3** Diseases that may mimic stroke

- Hypoglycaemia
- Todd's paresis following a fit
- Meningitis (p. 204)
- Encephalitis (p. 210)
- Cerebral malaria (p. 307)
- Brain abscess
- Brain tumour
- Chronic subdural haematoma (must be excluded by CT if there is a history of previous head injury, anticoagulant therapy or chronic alcohol abuse)
- Extradural haematoma (following trauma)
- Hypertensive encephalopathy (p. 135)
- Cerebral lupus

CT, Computed tomography.

■ **Table 27.4** Where is the stroke?

Location	Clinical features
Hemispheric	• Higher cerebral dysfunction (e.g. dysphasia) • Homonymous visual-field defect • Ipsilateral motor and/or sensory deficit
Brainstem	• Ipsilateral cranial nerve palsy with contralateral motor and/or sensory deficit • Bilateral motor and/or sensory deficit • Disorder of conjugate eye movement • Cerebellar dysfunction
Cerebellum	• Headache (usually occipital) • Dizziness, vertigo, nausea and vomiting • Nystagmus and gaze paresis • Truncal ataxia (may be unable to stand) • Limb ataxia (less common)
Lacunar Infarction*	• Pure motor hemiparesis • Pure sensory stroke • Ataxic hemiparesis (cerebellar and upper motor neuron signs in the same limbs) • Conscious level, higher cerebral functions and visual fields are normal

* Lacunar infarction is due to occlusion of a single perforating artery in the basal ganglia or pons by lipohyalinosis or microatheroma.

■ **Table 27.5** Potentially treatable causes of stroke

- Hyperosmolar hyperglycaemia (p. 259)
- Ruptured saccular aneurysm or AV malformation (p. 200)
- Cerebellar haematoma
- Embolism from the heart
- Aortic dissection and other extracranial arterial disease (p. 127)
- Vaso-occlusive crisis of sickle-cell disease (p. 299)
- Vasculitis (e.g. cranial arteritis)

AV, Arteriovenous.

2 Supportive treatment.

- Can the patient swallow safely? If the conscious level is depressed, oral fluids should not be given. If normal, test swallowing with sips of water taken with the patient sitting upright.
- If the patient cannot drink safely by 12–24 hours, start an IV or subcutaneous infusion (usually 2 l in 24 hours) or insert a fine-bore nasogastric tube. A speech therapist can give useful advice on the management of swallowing disorders.
- Start physiotherapy within 1–2 days to prevent contractures and pressure ulceration, and encourage recovery of function.
- Patients with language disorders should be referred for speech therapy.
- Give a stool softener to prevent constipation and faecal impaction.
- Urinary incontinence is common but often temporary: exclude faecal impaction and urinary tract infection. A urinary catheter (or penile sheath) should be used to prevent skin maceration.
- Deep-vein thrombosis is a common complication. The incidence can be reduced by early mobilization and graded compression stockings. Low-dose SC heparin may result in haemorrhagic transformation of a cerebral infarct and should not routinely be used.

3 Treatment of hypertension.

- Acute treatment is not indicated unless there is **hypertensive encephalopathy** (p. 135), **aortic dissection** (p. 127), or intracerebral haemorrhage with severe hypertension – systolic BP is > 200 mmHg or diastolic BP > 120 mmHg (for treatment see Tables 15.3 and 15.4, p. 134).

4 **Further investigation** is given in Table 27.6.

■ **Table 27.6** Further investigation of the patient with stroke

Blood tests

- ESR (? vasculitis, endocarditis, myeloma)
- Cholesterol and triglycerides in patients age < 50
- Syphilis serology (VDRL also positive in anticardiolipin antibody syndrome)

Urinalysis (? diabetes, vasculitis)

Imaging

Investigation sequence	Location of stroke		Brainstem or cerebellum	Severe stroke
	Lacunar	Hemispheric		
CT (not enhanced)*	Yes	Yes	Yes	Yes
Carotid ultrasound	No	Yes if good recovery	No	No
Echocardiography	No	Yes if carotid U/S normal and clinical evidence of cardiac disease	Yes if clinical evidence of cardiac disease	No

ESR, Erythrocyte sedimentation rate; CT, computed tomography; U/S, ultrasound.
* Cerebral infarction may not be evident on the initial scan and is best seen on a scan performed at day 7–10. Magnetic resonance imaging is better than CT at demonstrating lacunar infarcts and posterior fossa lesions.
Adapted from: Donnan GA. Investigation of patients with stroke and transient ischaemic attacks. *Lancet* 1992; 339: 473–7.

Secondary prevention

Applicable to all patients

- Cessation of cigarette smoking.
- Treatment of sustained hypertension.
- Dietary treatment of hyperlipidaemia.

Ischaemic stroke — no cardiac embolic source (haemorrhagic stroke excluded by CT)

- Aspirin 75 mg daily indefinitely.
- Patients who have made a good recovery from ischaemic hemispheric stroke should have carotid ultrasound to determine if they have a severe ipsilateral carotid artery stenosis for which endarterectomy may be appropriate (MRC European Carotid Surgery Trial, 1991; North American Symptomatic Carotid Endarterectomy Trial Collaborators, 1991).

Ischaemic stroke — presumed cardiac embolic source

- Patients with ischaemic stroke who do not have evidence of arterial disease, or who do have evidence of cardiac disease, should have echocardiography.
- The diagnosis of embolism from the heart is based on the presence of a cardiac embolic source, and associated features (Table 27.7).
- For patients with atrial fibrillation who have had a minor ischaemic stroke or transient ischaemic attack (TIA), the risk of further vascular events (especially stroke) is reduced by treatment with aspirin 300 mg daily or warfarin; warfarin is more effective (European Atrial Fibrillation Trial, 1993) if it can be given safely.
- Discuss with a cardiologist the management of patients with structural heart disease.

■ **Table 27.7** How certain is the diagnosis of stroke due to embolism from the heart?

Possible – the presence of cardiac embolic source

Major risk: atrial fibrillation; prosthetic valve; mitral stenosis; recent myocardial infarction; left ventricular thrombus; atrial myxoma; infective endocarditis; dilated cardiomyopathy; marantic endocarditis. These are associated with a substantial absolute risk of stroke, firmly linked to a cardioembolic mechanism

Minor risk: mitral valve prolapse; severe mitral annulus calcification; patent foramen ovale; atrial septal aneurysm; calcific aortic stenosis. These are associated with a low or negligible absolute risk of initial or recurrent stroke or are incompletely established as a direct embolic source

Probable – the presence of a cardiac embolic source and all of the following:

• None or minimal (< 50% stenosis) carotid artery atherosclerosis by ultrasound
• Non-lacunar infarct
• No other explanation for stroke
• No major cerebrovascular risk factor (chronic hypertension, diabetes)

Clinically definite – the presence of a cardioembolic source and either:

• Embolic occlusion on arteriography, without substantial proximal atherosclerosis; **or**
• Normal arteriography, with no other explanation for stroke and either non-lacunar infarct or lacunar infarct without chronic hypertension or diabetes

Reference:
Hart RG. Cardiogenic embolism to the brain. *Lancet* 1992; 339: 589–94, © by The Lancet Ltd.

Haemorrhagic stroke

• If primary subarachnoid haemorrhage (p. 200) is suspected (with focal signs because of extension into the brain), discuss further management with a neurosurgeon.
• Angiography may be indicated in a young patient with cerebral haemorrhage in whom an arteriovenous malformation is suspected: refer to a neurologist.

28 Transient ischaemic attack

Transient ischaemic attack (TIA) is defined as a focal neurological deficit of presumed vascular origin, which fully resolves within 24 hours (although deficits lasting longer than 1 hour are likely to be associated with some cerebral infarction).

Priorities

Your clinical assessment and investigation (Fig. 28.1 and Table 28.1) are directed at answering three questions.

Was this a TIA?

- The symptoms of TIA are of sudden onset, occur without prodromal features such as nausea or palpitation, reach their peak within seconds, and usually last for less than 15 min.
- TIAs usually cause loss of function; 'positive' symptoms (e.g. limb movement, paraesthesiae or visual hallucinations) are more likely to be due to epilepsy or migraine.
- Presyncope or syncope (p. 61) should not be attributed to TIA unless associated with other focal neurological symptoms.
- Other causes of transient neurological and visual symptoms are given in Table 28.2.

Which arterial territory was affected: carotid or vertebrobasilar (Table 28.3)?

- A carotid bruit is not a sensitive or specific sign of severe carotid artery stenosis.
- Carotid ultrasound is indicated in patients who have had carotid territory TIA and who would be candidates for carotid endarterectomy.

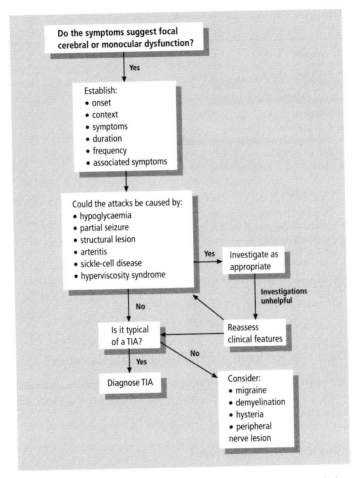

Fig. 28.1 Diagnosis of transient ischaemic attack. From Dennis M. *Hospital Update*. Dec 1991. 978.

■ **Table 28.1** Investigation of the patient with suspected transient ischaemic attack

All patients

- Full blood count
- ESR
- Urea, sodium and potassium
- Urinalysis
- Blood glucose
- Cholesterol and triglycerides in patients aged < 50
- ECG (? atrial fibrillation, LV hypertrophy, myocardial infarction)
- Chest X-ray (? lung neoplasm, cardiac enlargement)

Selected patients

- CT scan if there is doubt about the diagnosis of TIA
- Carotid ultrasound if carotid territory TIA (see Table 28.3)
- Echocardiography if carotid ultrasound normal and clinical evidence of cardiac disease

ESR, Erythrocyte sedimentation rate; LV, left ventricular; CT, computed tomography.

Does the TIA have a potentially treatable cause?

- Always consider **embolism from the heart**, **arteritis** (especially giant-cell arteritis (p. 75) in patients with transient visual loss), and **haematological disease**.

Further management

1 Further management of definite TIA is the same as that of minor ischaemic stroke (p. 189).

- If symptoms lasted > 24 hours, computed tomography (CT) should be done to exclude cerebral haemorrhage before aspirin is started.

2 If the diagnosis is unclear, refer the patient to a neurologist.

■ **Table 28.2** Causes of transient neurological or visual symptoms

Neurological

- Arterial disease: athero-embolism or arteritis
- Embolism from the heart
- Haematological disease: hyperviscosity syndrome, sickle-cell disease
- Migraine
- Hypoglycaemia
- Partial seizure
- Structural brain lesion causing focal epilepsy
- Compression of a peripheral nerve
- Multiple sclerosis
- Hysteria

Visual

- Arterial disease: athero-embolism or arteritis (esp. giant-cell arteritis)
- Embolism from the heart
- Haematological disease: hyperviscosity syndrome, sickle-cell disease
- Migraine
- Raised intracranial pressure
- Glaucoma
- Retinal detachment
- Hysteria

■ **Table 28.3** Symptoms of carotid and vertebrobasilar transient ischaemic attack

Symptom	Carotid TIA	Vertebrobasilar TIA
Dysphasia	Yes	No
Loss of vision in one eye only	Yes	No
Loss of vision in both eyes	No	Yes
Hemianopia	No	Yes
Diplopia	No	Yes
Dysarthria	Yes	Yes
Loss of balance	Yes	Yes
Unilateral motor loss	Yes	Yes
Unilateral sensory loss	Yes	Yes

29 Subarachnoid haemorrhage

Consider the diagnosis in any patient with:
- severe headache of sudden onset; or
- stroke with neck stiffness; or
- coma.

Priorities

1 **If the patient is comatose:** see Chapter 6 for initial management.

2 If the patient is not comatose, give pethidine (1 mg/kg) IM (plus an anti-emetic, e.g. metoclopramide 10 mg IM) to relieve the headache. The clinical features (Table 29.1) will usually allow you to distinguish subarachnoid haemorrhage from other causes of headache (p. 73).

3 **If the diagnosis is suspected, it must be confirmed or excluded by computed tomography (CT) or examination of the cerebrospinal fluid (CSF) (Table 29.2).**

4 If subarachnoid haemorrhage is confirmed, discuss further management with a neurosurgeon. Rupture of a berry aneurysm is the commonest cause **(Table 29.3)** and surgical obliteration of the aneurysm prevents rebleeding. The optimum timing of surgery is controversial.

Further management (before aneurysm surgery)

- **Bed rest**, preferably in a darkened side-room.
- **Drug treatment to reduce anxiety** may be helpful (e.g. diazepam 2–10 mg 8-hourly PO).
- **Analgesia** as required (e.g. codeine phosphate 30–60 mg 4-hourly PO). Start a stool softener to prevent constipation.
- Ensure an **adequate fluid intake** (3 l/day, giving some IV if needed).
- Treatment with the calcium antagonist **nimodipine** 60 mg 4-hourly

■ **Table 29.1** Clinical features of subarachnoid haemorrhage

- Severe headache of sudden onset – may be associated with transient loss of consciousness
- Nausea, vomiting and photophobia
- Conscious level may be depressed
- Neck stiffness – may be absent in the first few hours after a bleed
- Subhyaloid haemorrhages (retinal haemorrhages with curved lower and straight upper borders) – pathognomonic but uncommon
- Focal neurological signs if intracerebral extension
- Low-grade fever

■ **Table 29.2** Urgent investigation in suspected subarachnoid haemorrhage

Computed tomography

- Blood in subarachnoid spaces
- May show intracerebral haematoma

Lumbar puncture

- Raised opening pressure
- Uniformly blood-stained CSF
- Xanthochromia of the supernatant (always found from 12 hours to 2 weeks after the bleed; centrifuge the CSF and examine the supernatant by spectrophotometry)

Lumbar puncture:

- **should not be performed in patients with focal neurological signs or reduced conscious level** who may have an intracerebral haematoma
- **should be performed if CT is normal in patients with a suggestive history** (as minor bleeds may not be detected on CT); in order to confirm or exclude xanthochromia (the most reliable method of differentiating between SAH and a traumatic tap), lumbar puncture should be performed > 12 hours after the onset of headache, unless meningitis is suspected

by mouth or nasogastric tube (or by IV infusion via a central line: 1 mg/hour initially, increased after 2 hours to 2 mg/hour if no significant fall in BP) reduces cerebral infarction and improves the outcome after subarachnoid haemorrhage (British Aneurysm Nimodipine Trial, 1989). Nimodipine should be continued for 21 days.

■ **Table 29.3** Causes of subarachnoid haemorrhage

- Rupture of saccular ('berry') aneurysm of circle of Willis
- Bleeding from arteriovenous malformation
- Primary intracerebral haemorrhage with rupture of the haematoma into the subarachnoid space
- Bleeding tendency
- Bleeding from intracranial tumours, notably metastatic melanoma
- Trauma (most common in the elderly with occipital skull fracture)
- Unknown cause (i.e. cerebral angiography normal and no other cause identified)

■ **Table 29.4** Causes of neurological deterioration after subarachnoid haemorrhage

- **Recurrent haemorrhage** – peak incidence in the first 2 weeks (10% of patients)
- **Vasospasm** causing cerebral ischaemia or infarction – peak incidence between day 5 and day 14 (25% of patients)
- **Communicating hydrocephalus** – from 1–8 weeks after the haemorrhage (15–20% of patients)
- **Hyponatraemia**

Other therapies (e.g. with antifibrinolytic drugs) are not of proven benefit.

Problems

Hypertension

- First ensure that adequate analgesia has been given.
- If sustained and severe (systolic BP >200 mmHg, diastolic BP >110 mmHg) cautious treatment should be given. In patients not receiving nimodipine, start nifedipine initally 10 mg 8-hourly PO. Add a beta-blocker if not contraindicated, e.g. metoprolol initally 50 mg 8-hourly PO. In patients unable to take a beta-blocker, an alpha-blocker can be used, e.g. prazosin initially 1 mg 12-hourly PO.

Neurological deterioration (Table 29.4)

• Obtain a CT scan and discuss further management with a neurosurgeon.
• Check plasma sodium and urea: hyponatraemia may occur due to sodium depletion and/or inappropriate antidiuretic hormone secretion.

30 Bacterial meningitis

- Consider the diagnosis in any febrile patient with headache, neck stiffness or a reduced level of consciousness (Table 30.1).
- **If an intracranial mass lesion** (brain abscess or subdural empyema) **is suspected, computed tomography (CT) must be done before lumber puncture.**

Priorities

1 **If the patient is comatose:** see Chapter 6 for initial resuscitation.
2 **If the patient has septic shock (systolic BP < 90 mmHg):**
   - put in an IV line and give colloid 500 ml over 15–30 min.
   - take blood cultures and start antibiotic therapy immediately (see Table 30.3).
   - if you suspect meningococcal septicaemia (young adult with purpuric rash), give hydrocortisone 300 mg IV in case hypotension is due to adrenal infarction (Waterhouse–Friderichsen syndrome).
   - See p. 34 for further management of hypotension.
3 **If an intracranial mass lesion is suspected** (Table 30.2):
   - take blood cultures and start antibiotic therapy (Table 30.3).
   - Arrange CT scan.
4 **In other patients, a lumbar puncture should be done without delay** (p. 353). Record the opening pressure. Send cerebrospinal fluid (CSF) for cell count, protein concentration, glucose (fluoride tube), Gram stain (plus Ziehl–Nielson and India ink if immunocompromised: ? tuberculous or cryptococcal meningitis (p. 209).
5 **If the CSF opening pressure is > 40 cm, i.e. severe cerebral oedema, give mannitol 0.5 g/kg IV over 10 min plus dexamethasone 12 mg IV.** Discuss further management with a neurologist.
6 **If the CSF is cloudy, i.e. pyogenic bacterial meningitis, start antibiotic therapy (see Table 30.3).**
   - Adjunctive corticosteroid therapy may be of benefit in this group. Discuss this with a neurologist.

■ **Table 30.1** Neurological features of bacterial meningitis

- **Meningeal irritation:** headache, neck stiffness, vomiting, photophobia
- **Reduced level of consciousness**
- **Fits**
- **Cranial nerve palsies***

*** Long tract signs** (e.g. hemiparesis, extensor plantar response) suggest brain abscess or subdural empyema.

■ **Table 30.2** Features suggesting an intracranial mass lesion in the patient with meningitis

- Source of infection outside the central nervous system (e.g. middle ear or paranasal sinuses)
- Papilloedema (may also occur if meningitis is complicated by cerebral venous sinus thrombosis)
- Focal neurological signs other than cranial nerve palsies

■ **Table 30.3** 'Blind' antibiotic therapy for suspected bacterial meningitis in adults*

	First choice	**Second choice**
	Ampicillin 2 g 4-hourly IV **plus** Cefotaxime 2 g 4-hourly IV	Chloramphenicol 1 g 6-hourly IV

* Antibiotic doses must be modified in patients with renal failure.

- Intrathecal antibiotics are unnecessary and potentially dangerous.

Blood-stained CSF may be due to a traumatic tap or sub-arachnoid haemorrhage. Collect three consecutive tubes and check

■ **Table 30.4** Urgent investigation in suspected meningitis

- **Lumbar puncture** if not contraindicated
- **Blood culture**
- **Full blood count**
- **Blood glucose** (for comparison with CSF glucose)
- **Chest X-ray** (? pneumonia or lung abscess)
- **Skull X-ray** if suspected sinus infection (nasal discharge, sinus tenderness) or skull fracture
- **CT** if suspected intracranial mass lesion or skull X-ray abnormal

the red-cell count in the first and third. Check for xanthochromia in the supernatant by spectrophotometry (xanthochromia is detectable from 12 hours to 2 weeks after subarachnoid haemorrhage). See p. 200 for further management of subarachnoid haemorrhage.

7 Other urgent investigations in suspected meningitis are given in Table 30.4.

Further management

1 If organisms are seen on Gram stain, i.e. bacterial meningitis is confirmed: the cell count will usually be high with a polymorphonuclear leucocytosis but may be low in overwhelming infection.

- Modify or start antibiotic therapy (Table 30.5). **Obtain expert advice** from a microbiologist or infectious diseases specialist on the exact antibiotic regimen and duration of treatment.
- Adjunctive corticosteroid therapy may be of benefit in this group. Discuss this with a neurologist.

2 If no organisms are seen on Gram stain: management is directed by the clinical picture and CSF formula (Table 30.6).

- **Normal cell count, i.e.** meningitis excluded. Consider other infectious diseases that may give rise to meningism (e.g. tonsillitis, viral hepatitis).
- **High polymorph count.** This is typical of pyogenic bacterial

■ **Table 30.5** Gram stain of the cerebrospinal fluid in pyogenic bacterial meningitis

Appearance	Probable organism	Antibiotic first choice*
Gram-positive cocci	*Pneumococcus* *Staphylococcus aureus*†	Benzylpenicillin Flucloxacillin **plus** Rifampicin
Gram-negative cocci	*Meningococcus*	Benzylpenicillin
Gram-positive rods	*Listeria monocytogenes*	Ampicillin **plus** Gentamicin‡
Gram-negative rods	*Haemophilus influenzae* Enteric bacteria	Chloramphenicol Cefotaxime

* Dosage as in Table 30.3.
† For *Staphylococcus aureus* meningitis: (**a**) Flucloxacillin 2 g 4-hourly IV plus rifampicin 600 mg 12-hourly PO; or (**b**) Vancomycin 1 g 12-hourly IV (check levels) if methicillin-resistant *Staphylococcus aureus* infection is suspected or the patient is allergic to penicillin.
‡ Gentamicin dosage: see p. 84.

■ **Table 30.6** CSF formulae in meningitis

	Pyogenic	Viral	Tuberculous	Cryptococcal
Cell count/ mm^3	> 1000	< 500	< 500	< 150
Predominant cell type	Polymorphs	Lymphocytes	Lymphocytes	Lymphocytes
Protein concentration (g/l)	> 1.5	0.5−1	1−5	0.5−1
CSF: blood glucose	< 50%	> 50%	< 50%	< 50%

• The values given are typical, but many exceptions occur.
• Antibiotic therapy substantially changes the CSF formula in pyogenic bacterial meningitis, leading to a fall in cell count, increased proportion of lymphocytes and fall in protein level. However, the low CSF glucose level usually persists.

meningitis but may occur early in the course of viral meningitis. **If the patient has a reduced conscious level and/or CSF glucose is low, start antibiotic therapy.** If the patient is alert, the CSF glucose is normal and there are no other features to suggest bacterial infection, hold off antibiotic therapy and repeat the lumbar puncture in 12 hours. By this time an increasing proportion of the cells will be lymphocytes in viral meningitis.

- **High lymphocyte count.** This may be seen in many diseases (Table 30.7). Distinguishing between viral and partially treated pyogenic bacterial meningitis can be difficult. **If in doubt, start antibiotic therapy, awaiting the results of culture of blood and CSF.** If tuberculous or cryptococcal meningitis are possible on clinical grounds (Appendices 1 and 2) or on the results of CSF examination, ask for a Ziehl–Neilson stain and India ink preparation.

3 Supportive treatment of bacterial meningitis includes the following.

- Analgesia as required (e.g. paracetamol, non-steroidal anti-inflammatory (NSAID) or codeine).
- Control of fits: if fits occur, treat along standard lines with diazepam and phenytoin (Chapter 33).
- Attention to fluid balance. Losses are increased due to fever. Aim for an intake of 2–3 l/day, supplementing oral with IV fluids if needed. Check urea and electrolytes initially daily. Hyponatraemia may occur due to inappropriate antidiuretic hormone secretion (p. 267).

4 Contacts of patients with meningococcal meningitis should be

---

■ **Table 30.7** Causes of meningitis with a high CSF lymphocyte count*

- Viral infection
- Partially treated pyogenic bacterial infection
- Other bacterial infections – tuberculosis, leptospirosis, brucellosis, syphilis
- Fungal (cryptococcal) infection
- Parameningeal infection – brain abscess or subdural empyema
- Neoplastic infiltration

---

*Viral encephalitis (Appendix 3) may give a similar CSF picture.

identified. Rifampicin should be given to family members and other close contacts (600 mg or 10 mg/kg twice daily for two days).

5 The district community medicine specialist should be informed about confirmed cases of meningitis.

Appendix 1: tuberculous meningitis

- **At risk:** immigrants from India, Pakistan and Africa; recent contact with TB; previous pulmonary TB; alcoholics; IV drug abusers; immunocompromised.
- **Suggestive clinical features:** subacute onset; cranial nerve palsies; retinal tubercles (pathognomonic but rarely seen); hyponatraemia.
- The **chest X-ray** is often normal.
- The **CSF** usually shows a high lymphocyte count with a high protein concentration (see Table 30.6, p. 207). Acid-fast bacilli may not be seen on Ziehl–Nielson stain.
- **CT scan** commonly shows hydrocephalus (and may also show cerebral infarction due to arteritis or tuberculoma).
- Treatment: **combination chemotherapy with isoniazid, rifampicin, pyrazinamide and streptomycin.**
- Seek expert advice if the diagnosis is suspected.

Appendix 2: cryptococcal meningitis

- **At risk:** immunocompromised (organ transplant, lymphoma, steroid therapy, AIDS)
- **Suggestive clinical features:** insidious onset; absent or mild neck stiffness; papular or nodular skin lesions.
- The **CSF** usually shows a high lymphocyte count with a raised protein concentration (see Table 30.6, p. 207). Cryptococci may be seen on Gram stain as large Gram-positive cocci. India ink preparation is positive in 60%.
- The diagnosis may also be confirmed by CSF culture or **serological tests** for cryptococcal antigen on CSF or blood.

- Treatment: **fluconazole** or **amphotericin**.
- Seek expert advice if the diagnosis is suspected.

Appendix 3: viral encephalitis

- May be due to many viruses: **herpes simplex virus** is the most important as it may cause severe cerebral damage, which can be limited by early treatment with acyclovir.
- **Suggestive clinical features:** febrile illness, headache, personality change, abnormal behaviour, alteration in conscious level, fits, focal neurological signs.
- The **CSF** usually shows a high lymphocyte count (50–500/mm^3). There may be predominance of polymorphs in the early phase. Red cells are often present in herpes simplex encephalitis. The protein concentration is usually increased, up to 2.5 g/l. CSF glucose is usually normal but may be low. Save samples of CSF and serum for later assay of specific antibody titres, and repeat lumbar puncture in 10 days: a four-fold rise in **CSF viral antibody titre** is diagnostic.
- **CT scan** may show generalized brain swelling with loss of cortical sulci and small ventricles, but may be normal. In herpes simplex encephalitis there may be areas of low attenuation in the temporal lobes.
- **Electro-encephalography** (EEG) is usually abnormal in two-thirds of cases, with a spike and slow wave pattern localized to the area of brain involved.
- Seek expert advice if viral encephalitis is suspected. For suspected herpes simplex encephalitis, start **acyclovir** 10 mg/kg by slow IV infusion over 1 hour, 8-hourly for 10 days (reduce dose in renal failure).

31 Spinal cord compression

Consider the diagnosis in any patient with:

- **thoracic or lumbar spine pain;** or
- **weak legs but normal arms;** or
- **urinary or faecal incontinence.**

Early diagnosis and treatment are crucial to preserving cord function.

Priorities

1 **The working diagnosis of cord compression is based on the clinical features (Table 31.1).** The signs may be mild in the early stages.

- Details of the innervation of muscle and skin are given on pp. 400–403.

2 **Look for a cause:** cord compression is usually due to extradural disease (Table 31.2), of which malignancy is the most common.

3 **Obtain X-rays of the spine (Table 31.3):** these may show supporting evidence, but **if normal do not exclude cord compression.**

4 **Discuss further management with a neurosurgeon.**

- Magnetic resonance imaging (MRI) is the preferred investigation. Myelography should be performed if MRI is unavailable or contraindicated (because the patient has a pacemaker or is claustrophobic).
- If cord compression is due to malignancy, start high-dose dexamethasone (10 – 100 mg IV stat, followed by 4–24 mg IV 6-hourly; use the maximum doses in patients with severe or rapidly progressive signs, and lower doses if the signs are mild or equivocal). Further treatment is either radiotherapy alone or decompressive laminectomy followed by radiotherapy.

■ **Table 31.1** Clinical features of spinal cord compression

- Spinal or radicular pain
- Leg stiffness or clumsy gait
- Urinary hesistancy or frequency (painless retention is a late sign)
- Bilateral upper motor neuron signs in the legs
- Impaired sensation with a sensory level
- Reduced anal tone

■ **Table 31.2** Causes of non-traumatic extradural spinal cord compression

Cause	Comment
Malignancy	Most commonly carcinoma of breast, bronchus or prostate. Compression is at thoracic level in 70%, lumbar in 20% and cervical in 10%
Abscess	Severe back pain; local tenderness; systemic illness with fever
Haematoma	Complication of warfarin anticoagulation
Prolapse of cervical or thoracic intervertebral disc	
Atlanto-axial subluxation	Complication of rheumatoid arthritis

■ **Table 31.3** Urgent investigation in suspected spinal cord compression

- **AP and lateral X-rays of the spine** (look for loss of pedicles, vertebral body destruction, spondylolisthesis, soft-tissue mass)
- **Chest X-ray** (? primary or secondary carcinoma, tuberculosis)
- **Full blood count**
- **ESR**
- **Urea, sodium and potassium**

ESR, erythrocyte sedimentation rate.

Problems

The patient with known malignancy who has back pain but no abnormal signs

- With focal abnormality on spinal X-ray: discuss with a radiotherapist whether further imaging is needed before therapeutic irradiation.
- With normal spinal X-ray: arrange spinal CT or MRI.

32 Guillain–Barré syndrome (acute idiopathic polyneuropathy)

Consider the diagnosis in any patient with:
- **paraesthesiae in the fingers and toes;**
- **weakness of the arms and legs.**

Respiratory failure (which may rapidly progress to respiratory arrest) and **autonomic instability** are the major complications.

Priorities

1 Make the diagnosis from the clinical features (Table 32.1): generalized arreflexia is the clue (found in 75% of patients at presentation and 90% with fully developed illness). Other causes of acute polyneuropathy are rare and can be excluded on clinical grounds or by later investigation (**Appendix 1**).

- **Spinal cord compression** (Chapter 31) is the most important differential diagnosis, and should be suspected if there is a **sensory level** or **marked sphincter disturbance**.

2 Measure the vital capacity with a spirometer. Predicted normal values are given on p. 394. As a rule of thumb, vital capacity (ml) is 25 × height (cm) in men and 20 × height (cm) in women.

- **If no spirometer is available,** the breath-holding time in full inspiration is a guide to the vital capacity (normal > 30 s), provided there is no coexisting respiratory disease.
- **Arterial blood gases** can remain normal despite a severely reduced vital capacity and are not a substitute for measuring it.

3 Transfer to the intensive-care unit (ITU):
- **patients whose vital capacity is < 80% predicted;**
- **patients who are unable to walk.**

Discuss further management with an anaesthetist and a neurologist. Ventilation may be necessary (see **Problems** below). These patients are also at greatest risk of cardiovascular complications.

4 Admit other patients to a general ward for observation and further investigation.

■ **Table 32.1** Clinical features of Guillain–Barré syndrome*

- Symmetrical limb weakness proximal > distal
- Arreflexia
- Myalgia
- Bilateral facial weakness (in one-third of patients)
- Mild distal sensory impairment
- Absence of fever at onset

* **Miller–Fisher syndrome** is a variant seen in 5% of cases, characterized by ophthalmoplegia, ataxia and arreflexia with mild limb weakness.

Further management

1 **Confirm the diagnosis by cerebrospinal fluid (CSF) examination** which typically shows:
- **normal opening pressure;**
- **raised protein** (> 0.55 g/l after the first week of illness);
- **normal cell count or mild lymphocytic pleocytosis** (usually < 20 lymphocytes/mm^3 −2 > 50 makes Guillain–Barré syndrome unlikely, and other diagnoses should be considered).

2 **Electrophysiological tests** may be needed if there is doubt about the diagnosis: discuss this with a neurologist.

3 **Measure vital capacity (4-hourly–daily, depending on initial value)** until the weakness has reached a plateau.

4 **Plasma exchange** should be considered in patients seen within 2 weeks of the onset of weakness who need or are likely to need ventilation: discuss this with a neurologist. **Immunoglobulin therapy** may also be effective. **Steroids** and **immunosuppressive therapy** are not beneficial.

5 **Supportive treatment consists of:**
- Bed rest;
- physiotherapy to prevent contractures;
- ventilation for respiratory failure (see **Problems** below);
- Feeding by nasogastric tube (or parenteral nutrition) if lower

cranial nerve involvement interferes with swallowing;
- heparin 5000 U 12-hourly SC if unable to walk;
- aspirin or paracetamol for myalgia/arthralgia;
- stool softener to prevent constipation;
- fluid restriction if hyponatraemia occurs (due to inappropriate antidiuretic secretion).

Problems

Respiratory failure

- Patients whose vital capacity falls below 80% predicted should be transferred to the ITU with facilities for endotracheal intubation to hand.
- Measure vital capacity 4-hourly. As a general rule, ventilation is required if the vital capacity falls below 25–30% predicted.

Arrhythmias

- Transient arrhythmias (supraventricular tachycardia or brady-cardia) without haemodynamic compromise require no treatment.
- Severe prolonged bradycardias may occur and are treated with temporary pacing.

Abnormalities of blood pressure

- Sustained severe hypertension (diastolic BP > 120 mmHg) should be treated with labetalol by infusion (p. 134).
- If hypotension does not respond to IV fluids (guided by measurement of central venous pressure), treat with dopamine or nor-adrenaline infusion (p. 374).

Appendix 1

■ Table 32.2 Causes of acute polyneuropathy

Causes	Clues	Diagnostic tests
Guillain–Barré syndrome	• See **Table 32.1** • Infection in previous month **(Appendix 2)**	• CSF: raised protein, normal cell count
Acute intermittent porphyria	• Abdominal pain • Tachycardia • Vomiting • Drug exposure	• Urinary porphobilinogen
Toxin exposure	• Occupational history	• Toxicology
Polyarteritis nodosa	• Stepwise progression	• ESR • Muscle biopsy • Angiography
Diphtheria	• Children • No immunization • Palate involved first	

ESR, Erythrocyte sedimentation rate.

Appendix 2

■ Table 32.3 Infectious diseases that may precede Guillain–Barré syndrome

- Hepatitis A and B (may be asymptomatic)
- Mycoplasma pneumoniae
- Cytomegalovirus
- Epstein–Barr virus
- Campylobacter jejuni enteritis
- HIV

HIV, Human immunodeficiency virus.

33 Epilepsy

Major tonic–clonic status epilepticus

- Defined as a **generalized tonic–clonic fit lasting more than 30 min or repeated fits without recovery of normal alertness in between**.
- Prompt treatment is needed to reduce cerebral damage and metabolic complications (hypoglycaemia, lactic acidosis and hyperpyrexia), and prevent mortality.
- Consider the possibility of **pseudoseizure** if the clinical features are atypical (Table 33.1) and the patient has had previous admissions with pseudoseizure. If the diagnosis is uncertain, arrange an electroencephalography (EEG) during the attack. Check the serum prolactin: a normal level in a sample taken within 30 min of the fit supports the diagnosis of pseudoseizure.

Priorities

1 **Establish a clear airway, remove false teeth and give oxygen. Place in the lateral semiprone position.**

2 **Put in an IV cannula and give diazepam IV (Diazemuls), 10 mg bolus followed by a further 10 mg over 1–2 min.** Diazepam can be given by rectum (rectal solution – Stesolid) if an IV cannula cannot be placed).

3 **Take blood for stick test of blood glucose and the tests in Table 33.2. If blood glucose is < 5 mmol/l on stick test, give dextrose 25 g IV (50 ml of dextrose 50% solution), via a large vein.** In chronic alcoholics, there is a remote risk of precipitating Wernicke's encephalopathy by a glucose load; prevent this by giving thiamine 100 mg IV before or shortly after the dextrose.

4 **If the patient is known to have a brain tumour or active vasculitis, give dexamethasone 10 mg IV.**

5 **Unless the patient is known to be taking phenytoin with good compliance, give phenytoin IV 50 mg/min to a total dose of 18 mg/kg.**

■ **Table 33.1** Clinical features suggesting pseudoseizure

- Asynchronous bilateral movements of the limbs, asymmetrical clonic contractions, pelvic thrusting and side-to-side movements of the head
- Gaze aversion, resistance to passive limb movement or eye-opening, prevention of the hand falling on to the face
- Absence of metabolic complications
- No postictal confusion (drowsiness may be due to therapy given to treat suspected fit)

■ **Table 33.2** Immediate investigation in status epilepticus

- Blood glucose
- Urea, sodium and potassium
- Plasma calcium if hypocalcaemia suspected (recent thyroid or parathyroid surgery)
- Anticonvulsant levels (blood taken for later analysis)
- Arterial blood gases and pH

In the average adult, this comes to 1 g over 20 min. Attach the patient to an ECG monitor during infusion as phenytoin may cause arrhythmias (and may also cause hypotension if given too quickly).

Further management

1 If fitting continues despite diazepam and phenytoin: transfer the patient to the intensive-therapy unit (ITU) and **discuss management with an anaesthetist and neurologist**. Further anticonvulsant regimens may be tried:

- **chlormethiazole** (8 mg/ml) IV. Give a loading dose of up to 800 mg (100 ml) over 10 min (10 ml/min), and maintain with 0.5–1.0 ml/min (4–8 mg); or
- **phenobarbitone** 15 mg/kg IV, no faster than 100 mg/min or until

fits stop **only if the patient has not recently received oral pheno-barbitone or primidone**.

2 Correct electrolyte abnormalities.

• **Hyponatraemia:** if < 120 mmol/1, it should be corrected with hypertonic saline (p. 265).

• **Hypocalcaemia:** give calcium gluconate 1 g IV (10 ml of 10% solution) over 5 min.

3 Once fitting has stopped:

• Look for the cause (Table 33.3). Investigation is given in Table 33.4.

• **Seek expert advice** from a neurologist on maintenance anticonvulsant therapy and follow-up.

■ **Table 33.3** Causes of tonic–clonic status epilepticus

In a patient known to have epilepsy

• Poor compliance with therapy
• Therapy recently reduced or stopped
• Altered drug pharmacokinetics
• Pseudostatus (see Table 33.1)
• Intercurrent infection
• Alcohol withdrawal

In a patient not known to have epilepsy

• Brain tumour
• Brain abscess
• Stroke
• Meningitis
• Encephalitis
• Acute head injury
• Metabolic disorder: cerebral anoxia from cardiac arrest, acute renal failure, hyponatraemia, hypocalcaemia, hypomagnesaemia, hepatic encephalopathy
• Poisoning: tricyclics, phenothiazines, theophylline, isoniazid, cocaine
• Cerebral vasculitis
• Hypertensive encephalopathy

■ **Table 33.4** Investigation after control of status epilepticus or a first fit

- Blood glucose
- Urea, sodium and potassium (acute renal failure may occur after status epilepticus from rhabdomyolysis)
- Liver function tests, albumin and calcium
- Arterial blood gases
- Save serum (10 ml) and urine sample (50 ml) at 4°C for toxicology screen if cause of fit unclear
- Lumbar puncture if suspected meningitis (p. 204) or encephalitis (p. 210)
- Chest X-ray
- CT scan if acute head injury or conscious level remains depressed
- ECG (? long QT interval, conduction abnormality, previous myocardial infarction: if present, consider arrhythmia rather than fit)

CT, Computed tomography.

Single generalized tonic–clonic fit

First fit

1 Was it a fit or syncope? Distinguishing between a fit and syncope requires a **detailed history,** taken from the patient and any eye-witnesses (Tables 33.5 and 33.6). Common causes of fits are given in Table 33.7.

2 Your examination and investigation (see Table 33.4) are directed at establishing the following.

- Are there any **focal neurological signs**. Like an aura preceding the fit, these indicate a structural cause.
- Does the patient have an **infectious or metabolic disease** requiring urgent treatment, e.g. bacterial meningitis, acute renal failure?

3 If the patient is well:

- discharge if fully recovered and supervision by an adult for the next 24 hours can be arranged.
- advise the patient not to drive.
- outpatient investigation (EEG and cranial computed tomo-graphy (CT) if indicated) and follow-up by a neurologist should be arranged.

■ **Table 33.5** Was it a fit or syncope? Points to cover in the history

Background

- Any previous similar attacks
- Previous significant head injury (i.e. with skull fracture or loss of consciousness)
- Birth injury, febrile convulsions in childhood, meningitis or encephalitis
- Family history of epilepsy
- Cardiac disease especially previous myocardial infarction (at risk of VT)
- Drug therapy
- Alcohol or substance abuse
- Sleep deprivation

Before the attack

- Prodromal symptoms – were these cardiovascular (e.g. dizziness, palpitation, chest pain) or focal neurological symptoms (aura)?
- Circumstances, e.g. exercising, standing, sitting or lying, sleeping
- Precipitants, e.g. coughing, micturition, head-turning

The attack

- Were there any focal neurological features at the onset: sustained deviation of the head or eyes, or unilateral jerking of the limbs?
- Was there a cry (may occur in tonic phase of fit)?
- Duration of fit
- Associated tongue-biting or urinary incontinence?
- Facial colour changes (pallor common in syncope, uncommon with a fit)?
- Abnormal pulse? (Must be assessed in relation to the reliability of the witness)
- Any injury?

After the attack

- Immediately well or delayed recovery with confusion or headache?

VT, Ventricular tachycardia.

■ **Table 33.6** Clinical features differentiating vasovagal syncope from a fit

Feature	Vasovagal syncope	Fit
Occurrence when sitting or lying	Uncommon	Common
Occurrence during sleep	Uncommon	Common
Aura or warning • Duration • Features	Long Dizziness, sweating, palpitation, nausea	Short Focal central nervous system symptoms, automatisms, hallucinations
Pallor at onset	Common	Uncommon
Tonic–clonic movements	Uncommon	Characteristic
Tongue-biting and incontinence	Uncommon	Common
Injury	Uncommon	Common
Postictal confusion or headache	Uncommon	Common
Postictal paresis	Never	Sometimes (Todd's paresis)

Reference:
Schneiderman J. The first fit. *Med Int* 1992; 99: 4126–31.

- whether anticonvulsant therapy should be started after a first fit is controversial: find out the policy in your area.

Known idiopathic epilepsy
1 If the current history deviates from the usual pattern of seizures, consider:
- intercurrent infection;
- alcohol abuse;

■ **Table 33.7** Common causes of fits by age at presentation

Age 12–18	• Idiopathic epilepsy
	• Head injury
	• Arteriovenous malformation
Age 18–35	• Head injury
	• Poisoning
	• Alcohol withdrawal
	• Brain tumour
Age >35	• Brain tumour
	• Cerebrovascular disease
	• Alcohol withdrawal

   • poor compliance with therapy.
2 Take blood for anticonvulsant levels.
3 Discharge if fully recovered and with no evidence of acute illness.
   • Advise the patient not to drive.
   • Arrange outpatient follow-up before discharge.

Fit related to alcohol withdrawal

• Alcohol withdrawal fits – 'rum fits' consist of one to six tonic–clonic fits without focal features, which begin within 48 hours of stopping drinking and occur over a 6-hour period. They are usually brief and self-limiting.
• **CT scan is not needed if:** (a) history of alcohol withdrawal is obtained; (b) no focal features; (c) no evidence of head injury; (d) no more than 6 fits; (e) fits do not occur over a period >6 hours; (f) postictal confusion is brief.
• Admit for treatment of alcohol withdrawal (p. 69).

34 Acute upper gastrointestinal haemorrhage

This usually presents with **haematemesis** or **melaena** but should be considered in any patient with:

- **syncope**, especially with associated anaemia;
- **unexplained hypotension**;
- **hepatic encephalopathy** (Chapter 35).

Inform the surgeons promptly about patients with major upper gastrointestinal (GI) haemorrhage: their optimum management requires close collaboration between medical and surgical teams.

Priorities

1 Put in a large-bore IV cannula (e.g. yellow or grey Venflon). **Take 20 ml of blood for urgent investigations** (Table 34.1).

2 Estimate the volume of blood lost from the history and signs: pulse rate, systolic BP and skin perfusion (Table 34.2).

3 If there is hypovolaemic shock (systolic BP < 90 mmHg with cold extremities) follow the procedure below.

- Give oxygen and attach an ECG monitor.
- Rapidly transfuse colloid until the systolic BP is around 100 mmHg. If, despite 1000 ml of colloid, the systolic BP is still < 90 mmHg use grouped but not cross-matched blood. Save a sample of the transfused blood for a retrospective cross-match.
- Put in a central venous pressure (CVP) line and adjust the infusion rate to maintain the CVP around +5 cm water.
- Put in a urinary catheter to monitor urine output.
- Start transfusing blood as soon as it is available via a second IV cannula.
- Correct clotting abnormalities. If the prothrombin time is > 1.5 × control, give vitamin K 10 mg IV (not IM) and 2 units of fresh frozen plasma. If the platelet count is < 50 × 10^{12}/l, give platelet concentrate. Recheck the platelet count if > 4 units of blood have been transfused.

■ **Table 34.1** Urgent investigation in upper gastrointestinal haemorrhage

- Full blood count
- Group and save serum: cross-match 4 units of whole blood if there is shock, significant blood loss or haemoglobin < 10 g/dl
- Prothrombin time (if liver disease is suspected)
- Urea, creatinine, sodium and potassium
- ECG if age > 60 or known cardiac disease

■ **Table 34.2** Upper GI haemorrhage: evidence of significant blood loss without shock

- History of syncope in association with bleeding
- Persisting tachycardia (pulse rate > 100/min)
- Systolic BP < 100 mmHg
- Cool extremities
- Postural fall in systolic BP of > 20 mmHg (from lying to sitting)

4 In patients without shock, but with evidence of significant blood loss (Table 34.2) or haemoglobin < 10 g/dl:

- start an infusion of colloid;
- transfuse blood when it is available;
- correct clotting abnormalities (see above);
- put in a CVP line if age > 60 or suspected variceal bleeding.

5 If there are no signs of hypovolaemia, either heparinize the venous cannula or start a slow infusion of normal saline to keep it patent.

6 Patients with suspected bleeding oesophageal varices constitute a special group. Urgent endoscopy is required, as endoscopic sclerotherapy is the main treatment; around one-third of patients with suspected variceal bleeding do not have varices. Management is summarized in Table 34.3. **Obtain expert advice** from a gastro-enterologist.

■ **Table 34.3** Management of bleeding oesophageal varices

- Ask for help from a gastroenterologist
- Correct hypovolaemia and clotting abnormalities
- Start a vasopressin infusion (via a central venous line). Add 120 U (6 × 1 ml ampoules, 20 U/ml) to 250 ml dextrose 5%. Infuse 50 ml (24 U) over 15 min and then 50 ml/hour (0.4 U/min) for 12 hours
- Give isosorbide dinitrate by IV infusion (to reduce the side-effects of vasopressin). Start at 2 mg/hour. Increase the dose by 2 mg/hour every 30 min to a maximum of 10 mg/hour provided systolic BP is > 90 mmHg
- If bleeding continues, insert a Sengstaken–Blakemore tube (p. 365)
- Arrange urgent endoscopy with a view to injection sclerotherapy
- Other supportive measures include sucralfate 1 g 6-hourly (orally or via gastric channel of Sengstaken tube) to prevent stress ulceration, and lactulose initially 30 ml 3-hourly to prevent encephalopathy (Table 35.4, p. 234)

Further management

1 Blood transfusion. This should be given until a normal blood volume has been restored as shown by:

- pulse rate < 100/min;
- systolic BP > 110 mmHg;
- warm extremities;
- urine output > 30ml/hour (0.5 ml/kg/hour).

If the initial haemoglobin was < 10 g/dl (indicating either prolonged acute or previous chronic loss), continue transfusion until the haemoglobin is around 12 g/dl. As a rough guide, each unit of blood restores about 1 g/dl to the haemoglobin count.

Check the haemoglobin daily for the first 3 days and again before discharge. If the final haemoglobin is less than 12 g/dl, give ferrous sulphate 200 mg 12-hourly for 1 month.

2 Allowed to eat, or nil by mouth?

- **Patients shocked on admission or with evidence of significant blood loss** should not eat until endoscopy has been performed, in case urgent surgery is needed.

■ **Table 34.4** Indications for sugery in patients with bleeding from peptic ulcer

Age > 60

- Continued bleeding (requiring > 4 units of blood/colloid over 24 hours after initial restoration of blood volume); or
- One episode of rebleeding (with fall in BP); or
- Endoscopy shows active bleeding from the ulcer or signs of recent bleeding (adherent clot, visible vessel) and endoscopic haemostasis not possible

Age < 60

- Continued bleeding (requiring > 8 units of blood/colloid over 24 hours after initial restoration of blood volume); or
- Two episodes of rebleeding (with fall in BP)

- **Patients without signs of hypovolaemia** can eat (but should remain nil by mouth for 6 hours before endoscopy).

3 Drug therapy? There is no firm evidence to support the use of antifibrinolytic therapy or drugs to inhibit gastric acid secretion in patients with acute upper gastrointestinal bleeding.

4 Emergency endoscopy is needed for patients with:
- **shock on admission (but not before adequate resuscitation);**
- **continued bleeding or rebleeding;**
- **signs of chronic liver disease or known varices.**

In such patients it may be more practical to perform endoscopy in the operating theatre with the patient prepared for surgery.

Other patients should if possible be endoscoped within 24 hours of admission.

Management after endoscopy

Peptic ulcer

- Bleeding from a peptic ulcer usually stops spontaneously.
- The mortality is highest in patients over 60 who continue to bleed or rebleed, and may be reduced by endoscopic haemostasis or surgery (Table 34.4).
- Drug treatment to heal the ulcer (e.g. H_2-receptor antagonist, omeprazole) should be given. In elderly patients, long-term treat-

ment with a gastric antisecretory drug may be advisable to prevent recurrent bleeding.

- Treatment to eradicate *Helicobacter pylori* may be indicated: discuss with a gastroenterologist.
- Patients with gastric ulcers (some of which are malignant) should have endoscopy repeated at 6–8 weeks.

Erosive gastritis

There are two groups of patients:

1 previously well patients in whom erosive gastritis is related to aspirin, non-steroidal anti-inflammatory drugs or alcohol. Bleeding usually stops quickly and no specific treatment is needed;

2 critically ill patients with stress ulceration, in whom the mortality is high. Treatment consists of:

- sucralfate 1–2 g 6-hourly PO or nasogastric tube;
- correction of clotting abnormalities (see above);
- as a last resort, if bleeding is catastrophic, surgery with partial gastric resection can be performed but carries a high mortality.

Mallory–Weiss tear

Bleeding usually stops spontaneously and rebleeding is rare. If bleeding continues, the options are:

- surgery with oversewing of the bleeding point;
- tamponade using a Sengstaken–Blakemore tube;
- interventional radiology – either selective infusion of vasopressin into the left gastric artery or embolization.

Oesophagitis and oesophageal ulcer

- Treat with omeprazole 20 mg daily for 4 weeks, followed by a further 4–8 weeks if not fully healed.

Problems

Suspected upper GI haemorrhage with 'negative' endoscopy

In a significant proportion of patients, a first endoscopy does not reveal a source of bleeding.

• Discuss repeating the endoscopy especially if blood or food obscured the views obtained.

• Patients who presented with melaena only should be investigated for a small bowel or proximal colonic source of bleeding if no upper GI source is found (Table 34.5). A normal blood urea suggests a colonic cause of melaena.

■ **Table 34.5** Small bowel and proximal colonic sources of melaena

- Adenomatous polyp
- Arteriovenous malformation
- Meckel's diverticulum
- Angiodysplasia of colon
- Inflammatory bowel disease
- Haemobilia
- Aorto-enteric fistula (from aortic graft)

35 Acute hepatic encephalopathy (decompensated chronic liver disease and acute liver failure)

Consider the diagnosis in any patient with:
- **jaundice:** and
- **abnormal behaviour or reduced conscious level.**

The commonest cause of acute hepatic encephalopathy is **decompensated chronic liver disease** (Table 35.1). **Acute liver failure (fulminant hepatic failure)** is uncommon: in the UK, **paracetamol poisoning** (p. 99) accounts for around 50% of cases, and **viral hepatitis** for around 40%. Other causes are given in Appendix 1.

Priorities

1 Check blood glucose by stick test. If < 3.5 mmol/l, give 50 ml of 50% dextrose IV. Start an IV infusion of 10% dextrose (initially 1 l 12-hourly) in all cases because of the high risk of hypoglycaemia. Use a large peripheral vein as it can cause thrombophlebitis. Recheck blood glucose 1–4 hourly.

2 Other investigations needed urgently are given in Table 35.2. **A prolonged prothrombin time** confirms the diagnosis.

3 If there is grade 3 or 4 coma (Table 35.3), transfer the patient to the intensive-therapy unit (ITU) for further management, which will include elective endotracheal intubation and ventilation.

4 Obtain expert advice from a gastroenterologist if you suspect acute liver failure or the patient has decompensated chronic liver disease with encephalopathy more severe than grade 2.

5 If acute liver failure is due to paracetamol poisoning and the patient has not already received **acetylcysteine**, this should be given using the standard regimen (p. 102), as it has been shown to improve outcome.

■ **Table 35.1** Causes of decompensation in chronic liver disease

- Acute gastrointestinal haemorrhage
- Drugs: diuretics, hypnotics, sedatives and narcotic analgesics
- Hypokalaemia, hypoglycaemia
- Intercurrent infection especially bacterial peritonitis
- Alcoholic binge
- Acute viral hepatitis
- Major surgery and anaesthesia
- Constipation

■ **Table 35.2** Urgent investigation in suspected liver failure

- Prothrombin time
- Full blood count (including platelets)
- Urea,* creatinine, sodium and potassium
- Blood glucose
- Paracetamol level
- Arterial blood gases and pH
- Blood culture
- Urine microscopy and culture
- Microscopy and culture of ascites if present
- Chest X-ray

For later analysis (if suspected acute liver failure)

- Liver function tests
- Markers of viral hepatitis
- Plasma ceruloplasmin in patients aged < 50 (to exclude Wilson's disease)
- Serum (10 ml) and urine (50 ml) for toxicological analysis if needed

*Urea may be low because of reduced hepatic synthesis; if markedly elevated with a normal creatinine, suspect upper gastrointestinal haemorrhage.

Further management of decompensated chronic liver disease

1 **Look for and treat precipitants** (see Table 35.1).

- **Spontaneous bacterial peritonitis** is common and may not be

■ **Table 35.3** Grading of hepatic encephalopathy

Grade 1 Mildly drowsy with impaired concentration and psychomotor function

Grade 2 Confused, but able to answer questions

Grade 3 Very drowsy and able to respond only to simple commands; incoherent and agitated

Grade 4 Unrousable: 4a, responsive to painful stimuli; 4b, unresponsive

accompanied by abdominal tenderness. If there is ascites, aspirate 10 ml for microscopy and culture. Assume peritonitis is present if ascitic fluid shows > 250 white blood cells/mm^3 of which $> 75\%$ are polymorphs, and treat with a combination of amoxycillin, gentamicin (p. 84) and metronidazole.

● Start 'blind' antibiotic therapy (p. 80) if there is fever, even in the absence of focal signs of infection.

2 Start a liver failure regimen (Table 35.4).

Further management of acute liver failure before transfer

Monitoring and general care

● Nurse the patient with 20° head-up tilt in a quiet area of an intensive-care unit or high-dependency unit, avoiding unnecessary disturbance.

● Monitor the conscious level 1–4-hourly, pulse and blood pressure 1–4-hourly and temperature 8-hourly.

● Check blood glucose by stick test 1–4-hourly and immediately if the conscious level deteriorates.

● Monitor blood oxygen saturation by pulse oximeter and give oxygen by mask to maintain $Sa_{O_2} > 90\%$.

● Give platelet concentrate before placing central venous and arterial lines if the platelet count is $< 50 \times 10^{12}$/l.

■ **Table 35.4** Liver failure regimen in decompensated chronic liver disease

Reduce the intestinal nitrogenous load

- Stop dietary protein
- Start lactulose 30 ml 3-hourly until diarrhoea begins then reduce to 30 ml 12-hourly
- Magnesium sulphate enemata 80 ml of a 50% solution 12-hourly (useful even in the absence of gastrointestinal bleeding)
- Neomycin may be helpful, although its contribution is controversial

Parenteral nutrition should be considered: it should be started early to prevent a hypercatabolic state

Reduce the risk of gastric stress ulceration

- Prophylaxis with ranitidine 50 mg 8-hourly IV or 150 mg 12-hourly by mouth or nasogastric tube, or sucralfate 1 g 6-hourly by mouth or nasogastric tube

Maintain blood glucose > 3.5 mmol/l

- Give dextrose 10% by IV infusion initially 1 l 12-hourly
- Check blood glucose 1–4 hourly and immediately if conscious level deteriorates

Fluid and electrolyte balance

- Low salt diet
- Potassium supplements to maintain plasma level > 3.5 mmol/l
- If IV fluid is needed, use albumin solution or dextrose 5% or 10%; avoid saline
- Treat ascites with spironolactone combined with a loop diuretic if necessary, aiming for weight loss of 0.5 kg/day. If refractory, use paracentesis with IV infusion of albumin

Drugs

- Give vitamin K 10 mg IV (not IM) and folic acid 10 mg PO once daily
- Avoid sedatives and opiates
- Other drugs that are contraindicated are listed in the *British National Formulary*

- If encephalopathy is grade 2 or more, or if systolic BP is < 90 mmHg, put in a pulmonary artery catheter (as the central venous pressure (CVP) may not be an adequate guide to left ventricular filling pressure), a radial arterial line and urinary catheter.
- Give blood if haemoglobin is < 10 g/dl. Fluid therapy should be with albumin solution or dextrose 5% or 10%. Saline should not be used.
- If encephalopathy progresses to grade 3 or 4, arrange elective endotracheal intubation and ventilation.
- Put in a nasogastric tube for gastric drainage if the patient is vomiting or is ventilated.

Management of complications

This is summarized in Table 35.5. **Cerebral oedema** occurs in 75–80% of patients with grade 4 encephalopathy and is often fatal. It may result in paroxysmal hypertension, dilated pupils, sustained ankle clonus and sometimes decerebrate posturing (papilloedema is usually absent). If these occur:

- give **mannitol** 20% 100–200 ml (0.5 g/kg) IV over 10 min, provided urine output is > 30 ml/hour and pulmonary artery wedge pressure is < 15 mmHg; check plasma osmolality – further mannitol may be given until plasma osmolality is 320 mosmol/kg.
- **hyperventilate** to a Pa_{CO_2} of 4.0 kPa (30 mmHg).
- If there is no response to these measures, give **thiopentone** 125–250 mg IV over 15 min, followed by an infusion of 50–250 mg/hour for up to 4 hours.

■ Table 35.5 Major complications of acute liver failure

Complication	Management
Cerebral oedema	See text
Hypotension	Correct hypovolaemia (aim for wedge pressure 12–15 mmHg) with blood or 4.5% human albumin solution. Use adrenaline or noradrenaline infusion (p. 374) to maintain mean arterial pressure > 60 mmHg
Renal failure	Correct hypovolaemia. Start dopamine infusion at 2.5 µg/kg/min (p. 385). Avoid high-dose frusemide. Start renal replacement therapy if anuric or oliguric with plasma creatinine > 400 µmol/l
Hypoglycaemia	Give dextrose 10% IV 1 l 12-hourly. Check blood glucose 1–4-hourly and give stat doses of dextrose 25 g IV if < 3.5 mmol/l
Coagulopathy	Give vitamin K 10 mg IV daily. Give platelet transfusion if count < 50×10^9/l. Give fresh frozen plasma only if there is active bleeding
Gastric stress ulceration	Prophylaxis with ranitidine 50 mg 8-hourly IV or 150 mg 12-hourly by nasogastric tube, or sucralfate 1 g 6-hourly by nasogastric tube
Hypoxia	Many possible causes: inhalation, infection, pulmonary oedema, atelectasis, intrapulmonary haemorrhage. Increase inspired oxygen. Ventilate with positive end-expiratory pressure if SaO_2 remains < 90%
Infection	Daily culture of blood, sputum and urine. Early treatment of presumed infection with broad-spectrum antibiotic therapy. Consider antifungal therapy with amphotericin if fever with negative blood cultures

Appendix 1: principal causes of acute liver failure

■ Table 35.6 Principal causes of acute liver failure

Cause	Agent responsible
Viral hepatitis	Hepatitis A, B, C, D or E virus; herpes simplex virus (usually associated with immunosuppressive therapy)
Drug-related	Paracetamol poisoning (p. 99); idiosyncratic reactions
Toxins	Carbon tetrachloride; Amanita phalloides; phosphorus
Vascular	Veno-occlusive disease; Budd—Chiari syndrome; heatstroke; ischaemia due to cardiac disease
Others	Wilson's disease; acute fatty liver of pregnancy; Reye's syndrome; malignant infiltration

36 Acute renal failure

The diagnosis is made from:
- a rapidly rising plasma urea or creatinine; or
- a urine output of < 400 ml/day or < 30 ml/hour for 3 consecutive hours – this is not an invariable feature and 'non-oliguric' renal failure may occur.

Causes of acute renal failure are given in Appendices 1–3: 'prerenal' causes are the commonest.

Priorities

1 Clinical assessment and investigation (Table 36.1) are directed to answering two questions.
- Is there a reversible cause (Table 36.2)?
- Is dialysis needed urgently (Table 36.3)?

2 Assess the patient's fluid status and put in a central line to measure the central venous pressure (CVP).
- Check the fluid balance and weight charts.
- Examine the patient for signs of volume depletion (JVP not visible, postural hypotension) or overload (JVP raised, peripheral oedema, basal lung crackles).
- Check the chest X-ray for pulmonary oedema.

3 If the patient does not have pulmonary oedema, give a fluid challenge (see Fig. 3.2, p. 37).

4 If systolic BP remains < 90 mmHg despite a positive fluid challenge (CVP increased > 2 cm water in response to 250 ml colloid over 15 min), start inotropic/vasopressor therapy (p. 40).

5 If arterial pH is < 7.0, give sodium bicarbonate 50 mmol (50 ml of 8.4% solution) IV over 15 min.

6 Is plasma potassium high?
- If it is 5.5–6.5 mmol/l, start calcium resonium (15 g 8-hourly PO).

■ **Table 36.1** Urgent investigation in suspected oliguric acute renal failure

- Plasma sodium, potassium, urea, creatinine and glucose
- Urine stick test, microscopy (see Table 36.5), biochemistry (see Table 36.6) and culture
- Arterial blood gases and pH
- Chest X-ray
- ECG

Abdominal ultrasound to exclude urinary tract obstruction may be needed urgently in certain clinical settings, e.g. after surgery which might have led to ureteric obstruction.

■ **Table 36.2** Potentially reversible causes to be considered in all patients with renal failure

- Hypovolaemia
- Heart failure
- Sepsis
- Hypotension
- Accelerated-phase hypertension
- Hypercalcaemia
- Nephrotoxic drug or poison (Appendix 2)
- Urinary tract infection (esp. of single kidney)
- Urinary tract obstruction

■ **Table 36.3** Indications for urgent dialysis in acute renal failure

- Hyperkalaemia refractory to treatment (see Table 36.4)
- Pulmonary oedema
- Severe and worsening metabolic acidosis

- **If it is > 6.5 mmol/l, treat as in Table 36.4.**

7 Insert a bladder catheter (with scrupulous sterile technique) and collect a specimen of urine for stick test, microscopy (Table 36.5), biochemistry (Table 36.6), and culture.

■ **Table 36.4** Urgent treatment of hyperkalaemia (plasma potassium > 6.5 mmol/l)

If the ECG has abnormalities associated with hyperkalaemia (widening of the QRS complex, loss of the P wave, peaking of the T wave or a sine wave pattern):
- **give 10 ml of calcium chloride 10% IV over 5 min.** This can be repeated every 5 min up to a total dose of 40 ml
- **give sodium bicarbonate 50 mmol (50 ml of 8.4% solution) IV over 15 min**
- **give 25 g of dextrose (50 ml of dextrose 50%) with 10 U of soluble insulin IV over 15–30 min.** This will usually reduce plasma potassium for several hours

If the ECG is normal, give dextrose/insulin alone

Further treatment is needed. Start calcium resonium and discuss with your renal unit: urgent dialysis may be indicated

■ **Table 36.5** Urinalysis and urine microscopy in acute renal failure*

Red cells, red-cell casts, proteinuria (+2 or more)
- Acute glomerulonephritis (Appendix 3)
- Acute vasculitis

Stick test positive for blood, but no red cells on microscopy
- Rhabdomyolysis

Tubular cell casts, granular casts, tubular cells
- Acute tubular necrosis

Normal or near-normal
- Pre-renal causes
- Urinary tract obstruction
- Some cases of acute tubular necrosis (more commonly in nephrotoxic or non-oliguric ATN)
- Hypercalcaemia
- Tubular obstruction
- Renal athero-embolism (consider in the elderly patient with renal failure and skin lesions (esp. livedo reticularis))

*ATN, Acute tubular necrosis. In patients with a bladder catheter, red and white cells in the urine may be due to the catheter itself.

■ **Table 36.6** Urine biochemistry in oliguric renal failure

	Pre-renal	Oliguric ATN
Urine osmolality (mosmol/kg)	>500	<350
Urine sodium (mmol/l)	<20	>40
Urine: plasma osmolality	>1.5	<1.2
Urine: plasma urea	>8	<2
Urine: plasma creatinine	>40	<20
Fractional excretion of sodium (calculated as urine/plasma sodium divided by urine/ plasma creatinine)	<1	>3

ATN, Acute tubular necrosis.
NB: these indices assume previously normal renal function and may not apply in the following situations: **(a) diuretic therapy**—which increases urinary sodium excretion; **(b) after contrast media; (c) chronic renal failure; (d) the elderly**—in whom tubular function and concentrating ability may be reduced; **(e) acute glomerulonephritis and acute interstitial nephritis**—which may give a low fractional sodium excretion; **(f) diabetic hyperglycaemic states; (g) hepatorenal syndrome.**

Further management

Suspected pre-renal failure but no response to fluid challenge

1 Give frusemide and low-dose dopamine (Table 36.7). These may prevent progression to acute tubular necrosis or convert oliguric to non-oliguric renal failure, making management of fluid balance easier.
  • Omit frusemide if aminoglycosides have been used.
2 If oliguria persists, or urea and creatinine continue to rise, it is likely that ischaemic acute tubular necrosis has occurred. The management is now that of established renal failure (see below).

■ **Table 36.7** Frusemide and dopamine for suspected pre-renal failure unresponsive to fluid challenge

Frusemide

- Do not give until you are sure that the patient is fully hydrated
- Do not give if aminoglycosides have been used
- Give 250 mg IV over 1 hour by syringe pump
- If the urine output remains less than 40 ml/hour over the next hour, give a further 500 mg IV over 2 hours by syringe pump
- If the urine output increases, further doses can be given as required up to a maximum daily dose of 2 g or a continuous infusion can be started (30–60 mg/hour)

Dopamine

- Give 2.5 µg/kg/min (see Table 60.9, p. 385) via a central vein

Renal failure 'out of the blue'

1 Causes are given in Appendices 1–3 and investigations required are given in Table 36.8.

- Always consider the potentially reversible causes given in Table 36.2.

2 Consider a post-renal cause: this can be present even if urine output persists if there is a non-functioning kidney on the other side from the obstruction.

- Are there symptoms of bladder outflow obstruction and was there a large residual volume?
- Perform a rectal/vaginal examination to exclude a pelvic tumour causing ureteric obstruction.
- Arrange abdominal ultrasound.
- Discuss further management with a urologist if bladder outflow or ureteric obstruction is found.

3 Is there evidence of intrinsic renal disease?

- Has the patient received any potentially nephrotoxic drugs (Appendix 2) or taken any nephrotoxic poison?

■ **Table 36.8** Investigation in established acute renal failure

- **Full blood count and film**
- **Clotting screen** if the patient has purpura or jaundice, or the blood film shows haemolysis or a low platelet count
- **ESR**
- **Serum complement and other immunological tests*** if suspected acute glomerulonephritis (Appendix 3)
- **Serum and urine protein electrophoresis**
- **Plasma sodium, potassium, urea, creatinine, calcium and glucose**
- **Creatine kinase** if suspected rhabdomyolysis (urine stick test positive for blood, but no RBC on microscopy)
- **Blood culture**
- **Urine stick test, biochemistry (see Table 36.6), microscopy (see Table 36.5) and culture**
- **ECG**
- **Chest X-ray**
- **Abdominal ultrasound** to exclude urinary tract obstruction and assess renal size (small kidneys suggest chronic renal failure)

ESR, Erythrocyte sedimentation rate; RBC, red blood cell.
* Antinuclear antibodies, antineutrophil cytoplasmic antibodies (ANCA), antiglomerular basement membrane antibodies.

- Does the clinical picture or findings on urine microscopy (see Table 36.5) suggest acute glomerulonephritis (Appendix 3) or interstitial nephritis?
- **A renal biopsy may need to be done to establish the diagnosis if pre- and post-renal causes and infection have been excluded:** seek urgent advice from a nephrologist.

Management of established acute renal failure

Indications for urgent dialysis are given in Table 36.3. Renal replacement therapy is best started early (e.g. when urea is around 40 mmol/l and creatinine around 600 µmol/l). **Haemodialysis** is usually available only in specialist renal units, but many non-specialist intensive-therapy units (ITUs) can now provide **haemofiltration** which is adequate in many cases: discuss this with your ITU. **Peritoneal dialysis** (if transfer to a renal unit for haemodialysis or local haemofiltration is not possible) is described in Chapter 58.

Before dialysis is required, the patient should be managed as follows.

Fluid balance

- Restrict the daily fluid intake to 500 ml plus the previous day's measured losses (urine, nasogastric drainage, etc.), allowing more if the patient is febrile (approx 500 ml for each °C).
- The patient's fluid status should be assessed twice daily (by daily weighing and fluid balance chart) and the next 12 hours' fluids adjusted appropriately.

Diet

- Energy content > 2000 kcal/day (8400 kJ/day)
- Protein content 20–40 g/day
- Sodium and potassium < 50 mmol/day.

Potassium

- If plasma potassium rises above 5 mmol/l despite dietary restriction, start calcium resonium which may be given orally (15 g 8-hourly) or by retention enema (30 g).

Infection

- Patients with acute renal failure (ARF) are prone to serious infection especially pneumonia and urinary tract infection.
- Urinary catheters and vascular lines should be removed wherever possible.
- If the patient develops a fever, search for a focus of infection, take blood cultures and start antibiotic therapy to cover both Gram-positive and negative organisms (e.g. amoxycillin 500 mg 8-hourly IV plus flucloxacillin 500 mg 6-hourly IV, or a third-generation cephalosporin).

Drugs

- Make sure all drug dosages are adjusted appropriately: consult the section on drug therapy in renal impairment in the *British National Formulary.*

To keep on good terms with your renal unit
- **Contact them early** about patients with ARF — preferably before plasma creatinine is over 400 µmol/l.
- **Preserve forearm veins** as these may be required for dialysis. Try to take blood samples from one arm only. Where possible, IV infusions should be given into central veins.
- **Check hepatitis-B surface antigen before transfer.**

Appendix 1

■ **Table 36.9** Causes of acute renal failure

Causes	Examples
Pre-renal	
Hypotension	Cardiogenic shock, septic shock
True volume depletion • Gastrointestinal losses • Renal losses • Skin losses	 Vomiting, diarrhoea, haemorrhage Diuretics, hyperglycaemic states Burns
Third-space sequestration	Intestinal obstruction, pancreatitis, peritonitis
Oedematous states	Congestive heart failure, cirrhosis, nephrotic syndrome
Selective renal ischaemia	Hepatorenal syndrome, bilateral renal artery stenosis
Post-renal	
Urethral obstruction	Prostatic hyperplasia or carcinoma
Ureteric obstruction	Carcinoma of the bladder, prostate, cervix or large bowel Calculi, papillary necrosis Surgical accident Retroperitoneal fibrosis
Intrinsic renal disease	
Glomerular	Primary or part of a systemic disease
Vascular	Vasculitis Coagulopathy, e.g. haemolytic–uraemic syndrome
Tubular	Acute tubular necrosis due to ischaemia or nephrotoxins Tubular obstruction in myeloma or acute uric acid nephropathy
Interstitial	Drug-related acute interstitial nephritis Acute bacterial pyelonephritis

Based on Rose BD. *Pathophysiology of Renal Disease*. New York: McGraw-Hill, 1981; 56.

Appendix 2

■ **Table 36.10** Drugs and poisons which may cause or contribute to acute renal failure

Impairment of renal perfusion

- Diuretics
- Non-steroidal anti-inflammatory drugs (interference with intra-renal blood flow)
- Angiotensin-converting enzyme inhibitors (especially in patients with bilateral renal artery stenosis)

Nephrotoxic acute tubular necrosis

- Aminoglycosides
- Sulphonamides
- Rifampicin
- Contrast media (especially in patients with volume depletion or pre-existing renal impairment due to diabetes or myeloma)
- Paracetamol poisoning
- Aspirin poisoning
- Ethylene glycol poisoning
- Methanol poisoning
- Amanita phalloides poisoning

Acute interstitial nephritis (rash, eosinophilia, eosinophiluria)

- Many antibiotics
- Diuretics
- Cimetidine

Appendix 3

■ **Table 36.11** Major causes of acute glomerulonephritis (GN)

Low serum complement	Normal serum complement
Systemic diseases	**Systemic diseases**
• Systemic lupus erythematosus	• Polyarteritis nodosa
• Infective endocarditis	• Wegener's vasculitis
• Cryoglobulinaemia	• Henoch–Schonlein purpura
	• Goodpasture's syndrome
	• Hypersensitivity vasculitis
	• Visceral abscess
Renal diseases	**Renal diseases**
• Acute poststreptococcal GN	• IgG – IgA nephropathy
• Membranoproliferative GN	• Idiopathic rapidly progressive GN
	• Antiglomerular basement membrane disease
	• Immune-complex disease
	• Negative immunofluorescence findings

Reference:

Madaio P, Harrington JT. The diagnosis of acute glomerulonephritis. *N Engl J Med* 1983: 309: 1299–302. Reproduced by permission of *The New England Journal of Medicine*.

37 Overview of diabetic emergencies

- Urine should be tested for glucose in all hospital patients.
- Blood glucose must be tested in any patient with glycosuria, any ill diabetic and any patient with a clinical state in which derangements of blood glucose must be excluded (Table 37.1).

Glycosuria on routine testing

- Check the blood glucose either whilst fasting or 2 hours after a meal.
- Diabetes is diagnosed by a fasting venous plasma level > 8 mmol/l or a level 2 hours after a meal of > 11 mmol/l.

Hypoglycaemia

1 **If the patient is drowsy or fitting** (this may sometimes occur with mild hypoglycaemia, especially in young diabetic patients):
   - **give 50 ml of 50% dextrose IV via a large vein or glucagon 1 mg IV/IM/SC.**
   - recheck blood glucose by stick test after 5 min and again after 30 min.
2 **Consider the possible causes (Table 37.2).**
3 **If hypoglycaemia recurs or is likely to recur** (e.g. liver disease, sepsis, sulphonylurea excess):
   - start 10% dextrose at 1 l 12-hourly via a central or large peripheral vein;
   - adjust the rate to keep the blood glucose level at 5–10 mmol/l;
   - after excess sulphonylurea therapy, maintain the glucose infusion for 24 hours then tail off, but check blood glucose by stick test routinely for 3 days;

■ **Table 37.1** Clinical states in which derangments of blood glucose must be excluded

Clinical state	Page reference
• Reduced conscious level	53
• Acute confusional state	66
• Fits	218
• Suspected stroke	189
• Salicylate poisoning	97
• Metabolic acidosis	398
• Severe hyponatraemia	265
• Sepsis	78
• Liver failure	231
• Hypothermia	279
• Parenteral nutrition	

■ **Table 37.2** Causes of hypoglycaemia

Common

- Excess insulin
- Sulphonylureas – more common with chlorpropamide and glibenclamide than with tolbutamide or glipizide
- Alcoholic binge
- Severe liver disease (p. 231)
- Sepsis

Other

- Insulinoma
- Hypopituitarism
- Adrenal insufficiency (p. 272)
- Salicylate poisoning (p. 97)

4 If hypoglycaemia is only partially responsive to 10% dextrose infusion:
- give 20 or 30% dextrose via a central vein;
- if the cause is intentional insulin overdose, consider local excision of the injection site.

Blood glucose >11mmol/l

1 Check the urine or plasma for ketones. If $\geqslant 2+$, measure arterial pH.
2 Assess the conscious level and state of hydration.
3 The patient can now be placed in one of three groups (Table 37.3).
4 Further management is as follows:
- **diabetic ketoacidosis (DKA)**: see p. 253;
- **hyperosmolar non-ketotic hyperglycaemia (HONK)**: see p. 259.

Poorly controlled diabetes

- Insulin-dependent diabetes: modify the insulin regimen (see Table 38.7, p. 258), or treat with insulin infusion (p. 262) if there is significant intercurrent illness (e.g. sepsis, myocardial infarction).
- Non-insulin dependent diabetes: if there is significant intercurrent illness, treat with insulin infusion (p. 262).

■ **Table 37.3** Categorization of patients with blood glucose >11 mmol/l

	Glucose (mmol/l)	Dehydration	Ketones	pHa	Drowsiness
DKA	>15	++	+++	<7.2	++
HONK	>30	++++	+	>7.2	+++
Diabetes*	>11	−/+	− to ++	N	−

pHa, Arterial blood pH; DKA, diabetic ketoacidosis; HONK, hyperosmolar non-ketotic hyperglycaemia.
*Either poorly controlled or newly diagnosed.

■ **Table 37.4** Management of newly diagnosed diabetes (blood glucose
> 11 mmol/l)

Clinical state	Ketones	Glucose (mmol/l)	Management
IC	+ to ++	> 15	Insulin
IC	+	11−15	Recheck glucose and ketones in 2 hours
Well	−/+	> 20	Oral hypoglycaemic
Well	−/+	11−20	Diet alone
Well*	++	> 11	Insulin

IC, Intercurrent illness.
*The patient has mild DKA caught early before major fluid loss has occurred.
Insulin can be given as an IV infusion (Table 40.2, p. 262) or as a four times
daily SC regimen (p. 258).

Newly diagnosed diabetes

• Management depends on the **clinical state**, **ketone level** and **blood
glucose** (Table 37.4).

• Provided the patient is well and not vomiting, insulin therapy may
be started at home with the help of a specialist nurse: **seek expert
advice** from a diabetologist.

38 Diabetic ketoacidosis

- **Consider ketoacidosis in any ill diabetic**, particularly if there is vomiting or tachypnoea. Beware diagnosing primary hyperventilation (p. 186) without excluding diabetic ketoacidosis (DKA).
- **DKA should be excluded (by measurement of blood glucose) in any patient with confusional state, coma or metabolic acidosis.**
- **Causes** of DKA are given in Table 38.1.

Priorities

1 **Check blood glucose (initially by stick test).** A value of less than 10 mmol/l excludes the diagnosis. It will usually be over 20 mmol/l. Other investigations required urgently are given in Table 38.2.

2 **If ketones are low (trace or 1+), suspect hyperosmolar non-ketotic coma (HONK).** Treatment is similar, but there are important differences: see Chapter 39.

3 **Oxygen** should be given if Pao_2 is < 10.5 kPa (80 mmHg) on air.

4 **Start fluid replacement via a peripheral IV line.**
- If systolic BP is < 90 mmHg, give colloid 500 ml over 15–30 min.
- If systolic BP is > 90 mmHg give normal saline, 1 l over 1 hour.

5 **Insert a nasogastric tube** if the patient is too drowsy to answer questions: aspirate the stomach and leave on continuous drainage. Inhalation of vomit is a potentially fatal complication.

6 **Give insulin 10 U IV while an insulin infusion is being prepared** (Table 38.3).

7 **Arrange to transfer the patient to the intensive-therapy unit (ITU) or high-dependency unit.**

Further management

1 **Fluid replacement. Put in a central venous pressure (CVP) line to guide fluid replacement if:**

■ **Table 38.1** Causes of diabetic ketoacidosis

In patients with known insulin-dependent diabetes
• Inappropriate reduction in insulin therapy
• Infection
• Surgery
• Myocardial infarction
• Emotional stress
Presentation of insulin-dependent diabetes

■ **Table 38.2** Urgent investigation in suspected diabetic ketoacidosis

- **Blood glucose** (stick test and laboratory measurement)
- **Ketones** (stick test of plasma or urine with Ketostix)
- **Urea, sodium and potassium**
- **Arterial blood gases and pH**
- **Full blood count** (high white count may be due to acidosis, rather than infection)
- **Blood culture** (by separate venepuncture)
- **Urine stick test, microscopy and culture**
- **Chest X-ray**
- **ECG**

- systolic BP is < 90 mmHg; or
- plasma urea is raised; or
- the patient is known to have cardiac or renal disease (if the ECG suggests recent infarction, fluid replacement is best guided by measurement of the wedge pressure (p. 323).

A standard regimen is given in Table 38.4 but must be adapted to the individual patient.

- Reduce the infusion rate if the CVP rises > +10 cm water.
- The infusion rate must take into account urinary losses of salt and water which will remain high until the blood glucose is below the renal threshold (around 10 mmol/l).

2 Potassium replacement.

- Give none in the first litre of normal saline whilst awaiting the plasma level.

■ **Table 38.3** Insulin infusion in diabetic ketoacidosis using a syringe pump

1 Give 10 U soluble insulin IV stat while the infusion is being prepared

2 Make 50 U of soluble insulin up to 50 ml with normal saline (i.e. 1 U/ml). Flush 10 ml of the solution through the line before connecting to the patient (as some insulin will be adsorbed onto the plastic)

3 Start the infusion at 6 ml/hour

4 Check blood glucose by hourly stick test, and 2-hourly laboratory measurement, and adjust the infusion rate as below. Blood glucose will usually fall by around 5 mmol/l/hour

5 If there is no fall in blood glucose after 2 hours, check that the IV line is running and double the infusion rate. Recheck blood glucose after a further 2 hours and double the insulin infusion rate again if necessary

Blood glucose (mmol/l)	Insulin infusion rate (ml/hour)	IV Fluid*
< 5	0	Dextrose*
5–10	1	Dextrose*
10–15	2	Dextrose*
15–20	3	Normal saline
> 20	6	Normal saline

* Use 10% dextrose if significant metabolic correction is still needed (persisting acidosis or ketones more than 1+); otherwise use 5% dextrose. Give concurrent normal saline if still hypovolaemic.

- On average, 20 mmol are added to each litre of fluid, but **titrate according to the plasma level** (Table 38.5): **hypokalaemia is a potential cause of death in treating DKA**.

3 Bicarbonate. This should only be given if arterial pH is < 6.9 and systolic BP is < 90 mmHg despite fluid replacement.

- Give 1 ml of 8.4% sodium bicarbonate per kg body weight over 30 min and recheck arterial pH.

4 Antibiotic therapy.

- Bacterial infection is a common precipitant and complication of ketoacidosis and may not cause fever.
- Check carefully for a focus of infection, including an examination of the feet and perineum.

■ Table 38.4 Fluid replacement in diabetic ketoacidosis

1 Your fluid regimen must take account of:
- the likely fluid deficit
- the BP and CVP
- coexisting renal or cardiac disease

2 Start fluid replacement via a peripheral IV line:
- if systolic BP is < 90 mmHg, give colloid 500 ml over 15–30 min
- if systolic BP is > 90 mmHg give normal saline, 1 l over 1 hour

3 Then put in a central line to monitor CVP if appropriate (see text)

4 Give normal saline:
- 1 litre over 2 hours (no added potassium until plasma level known)
- 1 litre over 4 hours (plus potassium chloride according to Table 38.5)
- 1 litre 8-hourly (plus potassium chloride) until the fluid deficit has been corrected (as shown by warm extremities with a normal pulse and BP)

5 When the glucose is < 15 mmol/l change to dextrose:
- Use 10% dextrose if significant metabolic correction is still needed (persisting acidosis or ketones more than 1+)
- Otherwise use 5% dextrose
- Give concurrent normal saline if still hypovolaemic

NB: Hyponatraemia may occur in DKA due to osmotic shift of water, or as pseudohyponatraemia due to hyperlipidaemia (with milky serum). **Hypertonic saline must not be given.**

■ Table 38.5 Potassium replacement in diabetic ketoacidosis

Plasma potassium (mmol/l)	Potassium added (mmol/l)
< 3	40
3–4	30
4–5	20
> 5	Give none

■ **Table 38.6** Treatment of diabetic ketoacidosis: monitoring progress in the first 24 hours

Check hourly

- **Conscious level** (e.g. Glasgow Coma Scale: p. 60) until fully conscious
- **BP and pulse** rate until stable and then 4-hourly
- **CVP** until the infusion rate is 1 l 8-hourly or less
- **Blood glucose stick test**
- **Urine output**

Check 2-hourly

- **Blood glucose laboratory measurement** until < 20 mmol/l then check 4-hourly
- **Plasma potassium** until the infusion rate is 1 l 8-hourly or less
- **Arterial pH** until > 7.3 and then monitor ketogenesis from the urine ketone level

- A case can be made for giving antibiotic therapy to all patients. In the absence of an obvious focus, give **amoxycillin 500 mg 8-hourly IV plus flucloxacillin 500 mg 6-hourly IV**.
- If there is infection of the feet or perineum add **metronidazole 1 g 8-hourly PR** and obtain a surgical opinion.
- Changes can be made once the results of bacteriology are available.

5 Give heparin 5000 U 8-hourly SC until the patient is well enough to walk.

6 Put in a urinary catheter if no urine has been passed after 4 hours, but not otherwise.

7 Monitoring progress. A schedule is given in Table 38.6. Fluid balance, clinical observations and biochemical results should be recorded together on a flow chart.

8 Changeover from infusion to SC insulin.
- Continue insulin by infusion until urinary ketones are negative or only 1+ (usually at 24–48 hours).
- The patient may then take food with soluble insulin given SC. Continue the infusion for 1 hour after the first SC dose.

■ **Table 38.7** Establishing a twice-daily SC insulin regimen

1 Estimate total daily insulin dose from recent requirements
2 Give two-thirds total daily dose before breakfast and one-third before supper, each dose made up half of short-acting (soluble) insulin and half of intermediate-acting (isophane or zinc suspension) insulin
3 Check blood glucose before breakfast, midmorning, midafternoon and before bedtime, aiming for levels between 4–7 mmol/l
4 Adjust insulin doses as required

Unsatisfactory blood glucose	Adjust
Before breakfast	Evening intermediate-acting
Midmorning	Morning short-acting
Midafternoon	Morning intermediate-acting
Before bedtime	Evening short-acting

- Start with short-acting (soluble) insulin three times daily before meals and intermediate-acting (isophane or zinc suspension) insulin at bedtime. Base the total daily dose on double the total dose of insulin given over the last 12 hours.
- Check blood glucose 6-hourly and give top-up soluble insulin injections if it rises above 15 mmol/l.
- When insulin requirements are stable, change newly diagnosed diabetic patients to a twice-daily insulin regimen (Table 38.7). Put known diabetic patients back onto their usual regimen.

39 Hyperosmolar non-ketotic hyperglycaemia

Consider the diagnosis in the patient with hyperglycaemia where dehydration and drowsiness are severe.

Hyperosmolar non-ketotic hyperglycaemia (HONK) is differentiated from diabetic ketoacidosis by:

- blood glucose > 30 mmol/l, but only trace or $1+$ ketones in plasma or urine;
- plasma osmolality > 350 mosmol/kg (normal range $285-295$ mosmol/kg). This can be measured directly or calculated from the formula: plasma osmolality = [2(Na + K) + urea + glucose].

Management

This is the same as for diabetic ketoacidosis (DKA) with the exceptions below.

1 Half-normal saline is used for fluid replacement if plasma sodium is > 145 mmol/l.

2 Insulin sensitivity is greater in the absence of severe acidosis (Table 39.1).

3 The risk of thromboembolism is high. Unless contraindicated (e.g. recent stroke), start a heparin infusion (p. 386).

4 Total body potassium is lower and the plasma level more variable as treatment begins. Check the level 30 min after starting insulin and then 2-hourly.

5 Most patients can subsequently be maintained on oral hypoglycaemic therapy (or even by diet alone). Start an oral hypoglycaemic in place of insulin if the daily insulin requirement falls to around 20 U.

■ **Table 39.1** Insulin infusion in hyperosmolar non-ketotic hyperglycaemia using a syringe pump

---

1 Give 10 U soluble insulin IV stat while the infusion is being prepared
2 Make 50 U of soluble insulin up to 50 ml with normal saline (i.e. 1 U/ml). Flush 10 ml of the solution through the line before connecting to the patient (as some insulin will be adsorbed onto the plastic)
3 Start the infusion at 3 ml/hour
4 Check blood glucose hourly by stick test, and 2-hourly by laboratory measurement, and adjust the infusion rate as below. Blood glucose will usually fall by around 5 mmol/l/hour
5 If there is no fall in blood glucose after 2 hours, check that the IV line is running and double the infusion rate. Recheck blood glucose after a further 2 hours and double the insulin infusion rate again if necessary

Blood glucose (mmol/l)	Insulin infusion rate (ml/hour)	IV Fluid*
< 5	0	Dextrose*
5–15	1	Dextrose*
15–20	2	Normal saline†
> 20	3	Normal saline†

* Use 10% dextrose if significant metabolic correction is still needed (persisting acidosis or ketones more than 1+); otherwise use 5% dextrose. Give concurrent normal saline if still hypovolaemic.
† **Half-normal saline** is used for fluid replacement if plasma sodium is > 145 mmo/l.

40 Perioperative management of diabetes

The perioperative management of the diabetic patient is determined by the factors listed below.

- The **nature of the surgery** (**minor surgery** is defined as a procedure after which the patient may be expected to eat and drink within 4 hours; all other procedures are classed as **major**).

- Whether the patient has **insulin-dependent (IDDM) or non-insulin dependent diabetes (NIDDM)** (insulin-treated NIDDM is managed as IDDM).

- The **quality of preoperative diabetic control** (Table 40.1). Good control is defined as a random blood glucose on admission of < 10 mmol/l. If this is > 15 mmol/l, consider postponing non-urgent procedures so that control can be improved: **seek expert advice** from a diabetologist.

Insulin-dependent/insulin-treated diabetes

Minor surgery

This protocol is only suitable for patients whose **random blood glucose is < 10 mmol/l** on admission and are **first on a morning list**. Manage other patients as for major surgery.

Preoperative
Give usual medication.

Day of operation
1 Omit usual morning insulin if blood glucose is < 7 mmol/l. Give half of usual morning insulin if blood glucose is > 7 mmol/l.
2 Check blood glucose by stick test:
  - 1 hour preoperatively, i.e. at time of premedication;
  - at least once during the procedure;
  - 2-hourly until the patient is eating/drinking;
  - then 4-hourly.

■ Table 40.1 Preoperative assessment of the diabetic patient

- **Random blood glucose (laboratory measurement) on admission**
- **Blood glucose by stick test: (a) 4-hourly if insulin-dependent/treated;**
- **(b) 8-hourly if non-insulin dependent**
- **Urinalysis 6-hourly for ketones and glucose (throughout admission)**
- **Urea, sodium and potassium**

■ Table 40.2 Continuous insulin infusion using a syringe pump

- Make 50 U of soluble insulin up to 50 ml with normal saline (i.e. 1 U/ml). Flush 10 ml of the solution through the line before connecting to the patient (as some of this insulin will be adsorbed onto the plastic)
- Check blood glucose and start the infusion at the appropriate rate

Blood glucose (mmol/l)	Insulin infusion rate (ml/hour)
< 5	0
5–10	1
10–15	2
15–20	3
> 20	6 and review

- Check blood glucose at least 2-hourly and adjust the infusion rate as needed
- Aim to keep blood glucose between 5–10 mmol/l

3 Restart usual insulin regimen.
4 If blood glucose is > 10 mmol/l on two consecutive readings, set up an insulin infusion (Table 40.2).

Major surgery

Preoperative
Give usual medication.

Day of operation
1 Omit usual SC insulin.

2 Start an insulin infusion (Table 40.2).

3 Start an infusion of dextrose 5%, 1 l 12-hourly IV.

4 Check blood glucose by stick test:
- 2-hourly;
- at least once during surgery;
- each hour if surgery takes longer than 1 hour;
- at least once in the recovery area;
- 2-hourly postoperatively.

Postoperatively

- Continue insulin infusion until the patient is able to eat and drink.
- Continue dextrose 5% 1 l 12-hourly IV, plus additional fluids if needed.
- When the patient is eating and drinking, take down the insulin and dextrose infusions and restart SC insulin.
- The usual SC insulin regimen may need to be modified until a full diet is resumed: control may initially be easier using a regimen of short-acting (soluble) insulin given before meals and intermediate-acting (isophane or zinc suspension) insulin at bedtime (p. 258).

Non-insulin-dependent diabetes

Minor surgery

This protocol is only suitable for patients whose **random blood glucose is < 10 mmol/l**. Manage other patients as for major surgery.

Preoperative

Give usual medication.

Day of operation

1 Omit usual oral hypoglycaemic therapy.

2 Check blood glucose by stick test:
- one hour pre-operatively, i.e. at time of premedication;
- at least once during the procedure;

- 2-hourly until the patient is eating/drinking;
- then 8-hourly.

Major surgery

Preoperative
Give usual medication.

Day of operation
1 Omit oral hypoglycaemic therapy.
2 Start an insulin infusion (see Table 40.2).
3 Start an infusion of dextrose 5%, 1 l 12-hourly IV.
4 Check blood glucose by stick test:
  - 2-hourly;
  - at least once during surgery;
  - each hour if surgery takes longer than 1 hour;
  - at least once in the recovery area;
  - 2-hourly postoperatively.

Postoperatively
- Continue insulin infusion until the patient is able to eat and drink.
- Continue dextrose 5% 1 l 12-hourly IV, plus additional fluids if needed.
- When the patient is eating and drinking, take down the insulin and dextrose infusions and restart usual oral hypoglycaemic therapy.

41 Hyponatraemia

• **Consider the diagnosis** in any patient with **headache, nausea, vomiting or weakness. Late symptoms are confusional state, reduced conscious level and fits.**

• If a patient with an IV infusion has an unexpectedly low plasma sodium concentration, check first that the blood sample was not taken from a downstream vein.

• **Hyponatraemia is common in ill patients but only requires urgent treatment if causing severe neurological symptoms**, when plasma sodium concentration will be < 120 mmol/l.

Hyponatraemia causing severe neurological symptoms

Priorities

1 If the patient is comatose, start resuscitation along standard lines (p. 53). Fits should be treated with diazepam IV (p. 218).

2 Check blood glucose.

• **Hyponatraemia may occur in severe hyperglycaemia** due to osmotic shift of water from the intracellular space. Plasma osmolality is normal or high, and **treatment with hypertonic saline is inappropriate and may be fatal.**

• For further management of hyperglycaemic states see p. 253 (diabetic ketoacidosis) and p. 259 (hyperosmolar non-ketotic hyperglycaemia).

3 Assess the patient's fluid status from the fluid charts, BP, jugular venous pressure (JVP) and the presence or absence of peripheral and pulmonary oedema. Check previous biochemical results. Is renal function normal? Is cardiac function normal? How quickly has hyponatraemia developed?

4 If significant hyponatraemia is confirmed (plasma sodium

< 120 mmol/l), transfer to the intensive-therapy unit (ITU) for treatment (Tables 41.1 and 41.2).

Problems

Severe hyponatraemia in the patient with renal failure

Contact your renal unit. Treatment with hypertonic saline may precipitate pulmonary oedema, and dialysis should be used to restore plasma sodium to normal.

The comatose patient: when should hyponatraemia be treated?

• Treatment with hypertonic saline should not be given unless plasma sodium is < 120 mmol/l.

• If plasma sodium is $120-130$ mmol/l, other causes of coma should be suspected, e.g. subarachnoid haemorrhage or meningitis, liver failure, acute renal failure and diabetic emergencies.

Hyponatraemia without severe neurological effects

• If the patient has no symptoms attributable to hyponatraemia or is only mildly symptomatic (e.g. headache, nausea, lethargy), hypertonic saline should not be given.

■ **Table 41.1** Hyponatraemia with severe neurological symptoms: choice of treatment

Status	Treatment
Volume-depleted	**Isotonic saline IV**, guided by CVP measurement (p. 37)
Volume-overloaded or impaired cardiac function	**Hypertonic saline IV** (see Table 41.2) plus **frusemide IV**
Normovolaemic with normal cardiac function	**Hypertonic saline IV** (Table 41.2)

CVP, Central venous pressure.

■ **Table 41.2** Hyponatraemia with severe neurological symptoms: hypertonic saline therapy

1 The target is an increase in plasma sodium of 20–25 mmol/l or to 130 mmol/l, or relief of symptoms

2 Plasma sodium should be increased by no more than 1 mmol/l/hour (and no more than 25 mmol over 48 hours)

3 The hypertonic saline regimen needed is determined as follows
- Estimate the patient's total body water volume (litres) (the average value is 50% of body weight, but ranges from 35% of body weight in elderly obese women to 60% of body weight in young men)
- Subtract the patient's plasma sodium from 130: this number is the required correction of plasma sodium in mmol/l, and the number of hours over which plasma sodium should be corrected
- Multiply the total body water volume (litres) by the required correction of plasma sodium (mmol/l). This gives the number of mmol of sodium needed to correct the patient's plasma sodium to 130 mmol/l
- Divide the number of mmol of sodium needed for correction by 514 (the number of mmol of sodium in 1 l of 514 mM sodium (chloride). Multiply by 1000 to give the number of ml of 514 mM sodium chloride needed to correct plasma sodium to 130 mmol/l
- Divide the number of ml of 514 mM sodium chloride to be given by the number of hours needed for correction of the plasma sodium. This gives the infusion rate in ml/hour. Hypertonic saline should be given by a volumetric pump
- Give frusemide together with hypertonic saline if the patient is volume-overloaded or has impaired cardiac function

Reference:
Arieff AI. Management of hyponatraemia. *BMJ* 1993; 307: 305–8.

- Hyponatraemia is seen in a large number of diseases, usually late in their course when the diagnosis is obvious. However, it may be a diagnostic clue to several conditions (Table 41.3).
- SIADH – the syndrome of inappropriate antidiuretic hormone (ADH) secretion – is overdiagnosed. Inclusive criteria for the diagnosis are: **(a)** plasma sodium concentration < 130 mmol/l, plasma osmolality < 275 mosmol/kg, urine sodium concentration > 20 mmol/l, urine osmolality > plasma osmolality; **(b)** no oedema or signs of hypovolaemia (check for postural hypotension); **(c)** normal renal, thyroid

■ **Table 41.3** Diseases in which hyponatraemia may be a diagnostic clue

---

- Legionella pneumonia
- Adrenal insufficiency (p. 272)
- Hypothyroidism (p. 281)
- Diuretic or purgative abuse
- Acute intermittent porphyria (SIADH)
- Oat-cell carcinoma of bronchus (SIADH)
- Drug-related SIADH (e.g. chlorpropamide, carbamazepine, narcotics, chlorpromazine)

SIADH, Syndrome of inappropriate secretion of antidiuretic hormone.

and adrenal function (checked by Synacthen test); **(d)** the patient should not be taking diuretics.

Management

This depends principally on the patient's fluid status.

- **Volume-depleted:** give normal saline IV (with potassium supplements if required) until the volume deficit has been corrected. In asymptomatic patients in whom hyponatraemia is due to diuretic therapy, withdrawal of the diuretic and a normal diet is usually sufficient.
- **Volume-overloaded:** the combination of hyponatraemia and oedema can occur in congestive heart failure, liver failure, renal failure (acute or chronic) and the nephrotic syndrome. Correction of the hyponatraemia (if indicated) requires treatment of the underlying disease. Management is difficult and expert advice should be sought.
- **Normovolaemic (SIADH):** restrict fluid intake to 800 ml/day. In patients with oat-cell carcinoma of the bronchus, demeclocycline can be combined with water restriction.

42 Hypercalcaemia

- **Consider the diagnosis in any patient with unexplained non-specific symptoms** (anorexia, nausea, vomiting, constipation, thirst, polyuria, weakness, malaise, confusional state).
- **Severe hypercalcaemia** (total calcium > 3.0 mmol/l) is usually seen in patients known to have **malignancies involving bone** (carcinoma of the breast or bronchus, myeloma, lymphoma), but may sometimes be the presenting complaint. Much less often it is due to **primary hyperparathyroidism**.
- **Common precipitants** are dehydration, immobilization and treatment with thiazides.
- **Investigation** is given in Table 42.1.

Priorities

1 If plasma calcium is > 3.0 mmol/l and the patient is symptomatic, the first-line treatment is rehydration.
  - In patients with mild symptoms, oral rehydration (a fluid intake of at least 2–3 l/day) may be sufficient.
  - Patients with more severe symptoms should receive IV saline. Options are: **(a)** IV saline 3–4 l over 24 hours via a peripheral vein; **(b)** forced saline diuresis (Table 42.2): this is potentially hazardous and should only be used when rapid reduction in plasma calcium is required (e.g. because the patient is comatose or has major cardiac arrhythmias).

2 Peritoneal dialysis. Consider in severe hypercalcaemia complicated by renal failure: **seek expert advice** from a nephrologist.

Further management

1 If plasma calcium remains > 3.0 mmol/l despite rehydration, drug therapy to inhibit osteoclast-mediated bone resorption is indicated:

■ **Table 42.1** Investigation in suspected hypercalcaemia

- Full blood count
- Urea, sodium and potassium
- Uncuffed sample for calcium, phosphate, total protein, albumin,* alkaline phosphatase
- Chest X-ray
- ECG

If the cause of hypercalcaemia is not known

- Serum and urine protein electrophoresis
- Parathyroid hormone
- C-reactive protein and ESR
- Thyroid function tests

ESR, Erythrocyte sedimentation rate.
* Plasma total calcium should be corrected for the plasma albumin: add/subtract 0.2 mmol/l from the total calcium for each 10 g by which plasma albumin is below/above 40 g/l.

■ **Table 42.2** Forced saline diuresis for severe hypercalcaemia

- Put in a **urinary catheter** to monitor urine output
- Put in a **central venous line** to monitor CVP
- Give **normal saline** 1 l/2 hours IV
- Give **frusemide** 40 mg/hour IV
- If the CVP rises above +10 cm water, slow the infusion rate or give additional diuretic
- **Check plasma potassium and calcium 4-hourly.** Give potassium IV as required

CVP, Central venous pressure.

seek expert advice. The most commonly used agents are given in Table 42.3.

2 Specific treatment will be needed to prevent a recurrence of hyper-calcaemia (e.g. chemotherapy for malignancies, surgery for primary hyperparathyroidism).

■ **Table 42.3** Drug therapy in severe hypercalcaemia

Drug	Indication and dose
Pamidronate (biphosphonate)	**Indication:** agent of first choice in patients with non-haematological malignancy or primary hyperparathyroidism **Dose:** 30–60 mg IV as a single infusion or in divided doses over 2–4 days (in renal failure). Reconstitute each 15 mg with 5 ml water for injection then dilute with saline to a concentration of 15 mg in 125 ml. Give each 15 mg over at least 1 hour. Plasma calcium begins to decrease within 2 days and reaches its nadir within 7 days
Salcatonin (calcitonin)	**Indication:** failure to respond to biphosphonate **Dose:** 5–10 U/kg by SC or IM injection daily for 2–3 days
Glucocorticoid	**Indication:** treatment of lymphoma, myeloma, vitamin D toxicity and sarcoidosis. No response seen in non-haematological malignancy or primary hyperparathyroidism **Dose:** hydrocortisone 200–300 mg IV daily for 3–5 days

43 Acute adrenal insufficiency

- Consider the diagnosis in any patient with **unexplained hypotension or mild hyponatraemia and: (a) corticosteriod therapy** (prednisolone > 7.5 mg daily); **or (b) pigmentation** (buccal mucosa, scars, palmar creases); **or (c) preceding anorexia, nausea, vomiting and weight loss.**
- Causes of acute adrenal insufficiency are given in Table 43.1.
- Treatment requires **correction of fluid depletion** as well as **steroid replacement therapy**.

■ **Table 43.1** Causes of acute adrenal insufficiency

---

1 Rapid withdrawal of chronic corticosteroid therapy

2 Sepsis or surgical stress in patients with chronic adrenal dysfunction from:
- Chronic corticosteroid therapy
- Autoimmune adrenalitis
- Tuberculosis
- AIDS-related infection with cytomegalovirus
- Other rare causes, e.g. bilateral adrenal metastases

3 Bilateral adrenal haemorrhage due to:
- Fulminant meningococcaemia (Waterhouse–Friderichsen syndrome)
- Heparin or warfarin therapy

4 Sepsis or surgical stress in patients with hypopituitarism

Priorities

1 If the patient is unconscious, initial resuscitation is as for any cause of coma (Chapter 6). **Check blood glucose** by stick test: if < 3.5 mmol/l, give 50 ml of 50% dextrose IV via a large vein.
2 If systolic BP is < 90 mmHg, give colloid 500 ml IV over 15–30 min.
3 If acute adrenal insufficiency is possible, take blood for cortisol, and other investigation (Table 43.2) and give **hydrocortisone 100 mg IV**

■ **Table 43.2** Urgent investigation in suspected acute adrenal insufficiency

- Urea, sodium and potassium
- Full blood count
- Plasma cortisol (10 ml blood in a heparinized tube, for later analysis)
- Glucose
- Blood culture
- Urine microscopy and culture
- Chest X-ray
- ECG

Typical biochemical findings in acute adrenal insufficiency

- Raised urea
- Low sodium (120–130 mmol/l)
- Raised potassium (5–7 mmol/l)
- Low glucose

stat, followed by a continuous infusion of 10 mg/hour over the first 24 hours.

4 Start antibiotic therapy for suspected sepsis (p. 80):
- if the white count is > 20 or < 3 × 10^9/l; or:
- if there is fever or temperature < 36°C.

Further management

Fluid replacement

1 If systolic BP remains < 90 mmHg after 500 ml colloid, put in a central line and infuse colloid to keep the central venous pressure 5–10 cm water.

- **If systolic BP is > 90 mmHg**, give normal saline 1 l every 6–8 hours until the fluid deficit has been corrected, as judged by clinical improvement and the absence of postural hypotension.

- **Hyperkalaemia** is common in acute hypoadrenalism and potassium should not be added if plasma potassium is > 5 mmol/l.

2 Steroid replacement
- Continue hydrocortisone 100 mg IV daily until vomiting has stopped.

■ **Table 43.3** Commonly used corticosteroids

Steroid	Estimated potency	
	Glucocorticoid	Mineralocorticoid
Hydrocortisone (cortisol)	1	1
Prednisolone	4	0.25
Methylprednisolone	5	< 0.01
Dexamethasone	30	< 0.01

- Maintenance therapy is with hydrocortisone 30 mg PO daily which is given in divided doses (20 mg mane and 10 mg nocte) and fludrocortisone 50−300 μg PO daily.

3 To confirm the diagnosis in equivocal cases (where the initial cortisol level is borderline) and to differentiate primary from secondary hypoadrenalism, use the **short tetracosactrin (Synacthen) test**. This should be done when the patient has recovered, as hydrocortisone (but not fludrocortisone) must be stopped for 24 hours before the test.

Problems

The patient on long-term corticosteroid therapy (Table 43.3) or receiving replacement therapy. When should the dose be increased?

- **Mild infection** – double the usual dose.
- **Minor surgery** – 100 mg hydrocortisone IV 6-hourly for 24 hours starting with the premedication then return to usual dose.
- **Severe infection or major surgery** – hydrocortisone IV as for minor surgery but continue for 72 hours or until taking oral fluids. After this give the same dose orally (and restart fludrocortisone) and gradually taper over 2 weeks to the usual maintenance dose.

44 Thyrotoxic crisis

- Consider the diagnosis in any patient with **fever, abnormal mental state and signs of thyrotoxicosis** (Table 44.1).
- The mortality of untreated thyrotoxic crisis is high. If the diagnosis is suspected, **antithyroid treatment must be started before biochemical confirmation**.

Priorities

Clinical assessment

Clinical assessment is directed at:

1 making a clinical diagnosis of thyrotoxicosis (if this has not been previously confirmed by thyroid function tests); the signs may not be prominent in the elderly, or masked by other illness – check for goitre, thyroid bruit and ophthalmopathy;

2 identifying the precipitant (Table 44.2);

3 establishing the presence or absence of heart failure (raised venous pressure, basal lung crackles, peripheral oedema).

Investigations needed urgently are given in Table 44.3.

Supportive therapy

1 Treat sepsis (Chapter 10).

2 Treat heart failure. This is usually associated with fast **atrial fibrillation**. Cardioversion of atrial fibrillation is very unlikely to be successful until the patient is euthyroid: give **digoxin** to control the ventricular rate. There is relative digoxin resistance (increased renal excretion and reduced action on atrioventricular conduction) so high doses are needed:

- loading dose of 0.5 mg IV over 30 min followed by 0.25 mg IV over 30 min every 2 hours until the heart rate is < 100/min or up to a total dose of 1.5 mg;

■ **Table 44.1** Features of thyrotoxic crisis ('thyroid storm')

- **Fever** $> 38°C$, associated with profuse sweating
- **Agitation, restlessness and confusional state**
- **Tachycardia** (sinus tachycardia or atrial fibrillation)
- **Signs of thyrotoxicosis**

■ **Table 44.2** Precipitants of thyrotoxic crisis

- Infection
- Surgical stress
- Trauma
- Iodine: amiodarone; radiographic contrast media; radioiodine
- Pulmonary embolism
- Myocardial infarction

■ **Table 44.3** Urgent investigation in suspected thyrotoxic crisis

- Thyroid function (TSH, free T_3 and free T_4*) (for later analysis)
- Urea, sodium and potassium
- Full blood count
- Blood glucose
- Blood culture
- Urine microscopy and culture
- Chest X-ray
- ECG
- Arterial blood gases and pH

TSH, Thyroid-stimulating hormone; T_3, tri-iodothyronine; T_4, thyroxine.
* If severely ill, increased production of reverse tri-iodothyronine may lead to near normal thyroxine levels.

- maintenance dose of 0.25–0.5 mg daily PO.

Give **oxygen by mask** and a **loop diuretic** (frusemide or bumetanide) as required.

3 **If there is no heart failure**, give **propranolol** 40–160 mg 6-hourly

PO, aiming to reduce the heart rate < 100/min. **Diltiazem** 60–120 mg 6-hourly PO can be used if beta-blockade is contraindicated because of asthma.

4 Give **heparin** by infusion (p. 386) in patients with atrial fibrillation or if pulmonary embolism is suspected (p. 155). Other patients should receive heparin 5000 U 8-hourly SC as prophylaxis against venous thrombo-embolism.

5 Treat severe agitation with chlorpromazine (50 mg 8-hourly PO, or 25 mg 8-hourly IM, or by rectal suppository 100 mg 6–8-hourly).

6 Reduce fever by fanning, tepid sponging or paracetamol (avoid aspirin as it displaces thyroxine from thyroid-binding globulin).

7 Give **fluid replacement** guided by measurement of central venous pressure (CVP).

Antithyroid treatment (Table 44.4)

- Start either propylthiouracil or carbimazole (which act principally by inhibiting thyroxine synthesis).
- After 4 hours, start iodine (which inhibits secretion of thyroxine). If iodine is started before antithyroid drugs, excess thyroxine may be produced leading to an exacerbation of the crisis.

■ **Table 44.4** Antithyroid treatment in thyrotoxic crisis

Drug	Regimen
Carbimazole; or	15–30 mg 6-hourly PO/nasogastric tube, reducing to 10–20 mg 8-hourly after 24 hours
Propylthiouracil;	150–300 mg 6-hourly PO/nasogastric tube, reducing to 100–200 mg 8-hourly after 24 hours
plus **Iodine**	**Do not start within 4 hours of carbimazole or propylthiouracil.** 0.1–0.3 ml of aqueous iodine oral solution (Lugol's solution) 8-hourly PO/nasogastric tube. Stop after 2 days if propylthiouracil is used or after 1 week with carbimazole

• There is no evidence supporting the use of glucocorticoid steroids to reduce the peripheral conversion of thyroxine to tri-iodothyronine.

Exchange transfusion or peritoneal dialysis/haemodialysis

This may be considered in a patient who fails to improve within 24–48 hours. **Seek expert advice** from an endocrinologist.

45 Hypothermia (including myxoedema coma)

- Hypothermia is defined as a core temperature $< 35°C$.
- Coma occurs if the core temperature falls below $27°C$.
- Measure rectal temperature with a low-reading thermometer in any patient admitted with a reduced level of consciousness who has been exposed to the cold.
- At high risk are the elderly (in whom hypothermia is often the consequence of acute illness) and those living rough (often due to the combination of alcohol and cold exposure).

Priorities

1 **If unconscious, start resuscitation as for coma from any cause (Chapter 6).**

2 **Give oxygen, attach an ECG monitor and put in a peripheral IV line.**
- **Ventricular fibrillation** may occur at core temperatures $< 28-30°C$. Precipitants include central vein cannulation, chest compression, endotracheal intubation and IV injection of adrenaline. DC counter-shock may not be effective until core temperature is $> 30°C$. Continue cardiopulmonary resuscitation for longer than usual (as hypothermia protects the brain from ischaemic injury).
- Sinus bradycardia does not need treatment: temporary pacing is only indicated for complete heart block.

3 **Check blood glucose.** Treat hypoglycaemia. Raised blood glucose ($10-20$ mmol/l) is common (due to insulin resistance) and should not be treated with insulin because of the risk of hypoglycaemia on rewarming.

4 **Active rewarming** may be indicated if core temperature is $< 30°C$, or there is ventricular fibrillation (VF) refractory to DC shock: take into consideration the age of the patient and concurrent illness.
- See Appendix 1 for methods of active rewarming.

5 **Check for underlying illness** (e.g. pneumonia, stroke, myocardial infarction, fractured neck of femur) (Table 45.1).

■ **Table 45.1** Urgent investigation of the patient with hypothermia

- Full blood count
- Sodium, potassium and urea
- Blood glucose
- Arterial pH and gases (corrected for temperature*)
- Blood culture
- Thyroid function (if age > 50 or suspected thyroid disease) for later analysis
- Blood and urine for drug screen if no other cause for hypothermia is evident
- ECG
- Chest X-ray
- X-ray pelvis and hips if history of a fall or clinical signs of fractured neck of femur

* For each 1°C decrease in body temperature below 37°C, arterial pH increases by 0.015, PaO_2 decreases by 4.4% and $PaCO_2$ decreases by 7.2%.
Blood levels of skeletal and cardiac muscle enzymes are raised in hypothermia, even in the absence of myocardial infarction.

- **Consider poisoning with alcohol or psychotropic drugs** if no other cause of hypothermia is evident (Chapter 11).

6 **Is there evidence of myxoedema?**

- The physical signs of hypothermia from whatever cause closely resemble those of **myxoedema coma** (Table 45.2): however, if there is other evidence of hypothyroidism, thyroid hormone and hydrocortisone should be given (Appendix 2).

Further management

1 **Rewarming methods** are summarized in Table 45.3. Elderly patients are most safely managed by **passive external rewarming** (Table 45.4).

2 As **pneumonia** is a common cause and complication of hypothermia, give amoxycillin 500 mg and erythromycin 500 mg IV once blood cultures have been taken. Further doses need not be given until the core temperature is > 32°C.

■ **Table 45.2** Features suggesting myxoedema in the patient with hypothermia

- Preceding symptoms of hypothyroidism: weight gain with reduced appetite, dry skin and hair loss
- Previous radioiodine treatment for thyroxicosis
- Thyroidectomy scar
- Hyponatraemia (plasma sodium < 130 mmol/l)
- Macrocytosis
- Failure of core temperature to rise 0.5°C/hour with external rewarming

Slowly relaxing tendon reflexes are a non-specific feature of hypothermia.

■ **Table 45.3** Rewarming of the hypothermic patient

Core temperature (°C)	Rewarming methods
32–35	Passive external rewarming
	Hot drinks
30–32	Passive external rewarming
	Warmed IV fluids
	Warmed humidified oxygen
< 30	Peritoneal dialysis
	Cardiopulmonary bypass

■ **Table 45.4** Passive external rewarming

1 Nurse in a side room heated to 20–30°C on a ripple mattress with the blankets supported by a bed cage
2 Give warmed humidified oxygen by facemask
3 Aim for a slow rise in core temperature (around 0.5°C/hour)
4 Monitor:
- **rectal temperature** (hourly, or preferably using a rectal probe allowing a continuous display)
- **oxygen saturation** by pulse oximeter (continuous display)
- **ECG** (supraventricular arrhythmias (e.g. atrial fibrillation) are common and usually resolve as core temperature returns to normal)
- **BP** (hourly); if systolic BP falls below 100 mmHg, reduce the rate of rewarming and give further IV fluid
- **CVP** (hourly) (**NB**: do not put in a central line until core temperature is > 30°C as it may precipitate VF)
- **blood glucose** (4-hourly)
- **urine output** by bladder catheter (hourly)

3 Most hypothermic patients are **volume-depleted** (due in part to cold-induced diuresis). If the chest X-ray does not show pulmonary oedema, start an IV infusion of normal saline 1 l over 4 hours via a warming coil: further fluid therapy should be guided by the BP, central venous pressure (CVP) and urine output.

Appendix 1: methods of active rewarming

Peritoneal dialysis (See p. 360)

Inhalation of warmed oxygen (via endotracheal tube)

Oxygen is warmed in a waterbath humidifier. Monitor the gas temperature at the mouth and maintain it around 44°C (this will require modification of most ventilators).

Other methods

These include an **oesophageal thermal probe** and **cardiopulmonary bypass**.

Appendix 2: treatment of myxoedema coma

1 Check for concurrent illness.
2 Start antibiotic therapy with amoxycillin 500 mg 8-hourly and erythromycin 500 mg 8-hourly IV once blood cultures have been taken.
3 Standard management of hypothermia by passive external rewarming (see Table 45.4).
4 Take blood for thyroid hormones, thyroid-stimulating hormone (TSH) and cortisol before starting treatment.
5 **Thyroid hormone replacement**:
  • Start IV tri-iodothyronine (T_3) (Table 45.5). This has a shorter half-

■ **Table 45.5** Thyroid hormone replacement in myxoedema coma

Day 1–3	T_3: 10 µg 8-hourly IV
Day 4–6	T_3: 20 µg 12-hourly IV
Day 7–14	T_3: 20 µg 8-hourly IV
Week 3–4	T_4: 50 µg once daily PO

life than thyroxine (T_4) which is advantageous if haemodynamic problems develop and the dose has to be reduced.

• An alternative regimen is T_4 400–500 µg as a bolus IV or via a nasogastric tube. No further replacement therapy should be given for 1 week.

6 **Give hydrocortisone** 100 mg 12-hourly IV in case there is panhypopituitarism.

46 Acute medical problems in the patient with HIV/AIDS

- Human immunodeficiency virus (HIV)+ patients get common diseases as well as those that reflect their immune deficiency.
- Establish who knows the HIV diagnosis among the patient's relatives and friends and be sensitive to their needs.
- HIV+ patients have often made 'living wills': find out if one exists.
- Take appropriate safety precautions when handling any body fluid, and label all specimens as high risk (Table 46.1).
- When completing notifiable disease forms (tuberculosis, salmonella, hepatitis), HIV need not be mentioned. Acquired immunodeficiency syndrome (AIDS)-defining diagnoses (Appendix 1) should be reported to the Centre for Disease Surveillance and Control.

Breathlessness

*Pulmonary infection (especially with *Pneumocystis carinii*) remains the commonest acute presentation of HIV+ patients.

Priorities

1 Attach a pulse oximeter and check arterial blood gases: the patient may be severely hypoxaemic with minimal lung signs. Give oxygen to maintain arterial oxygen saturation >90%. Other investigations needed urgently are given in Table 46.2.

2 Your clinical assessment and the chest X-ray appearances may provide clues to the likely diagnosis (Table 46.3). Dual pathology is relatively frequent and definitive diagnosis depends on microbiological findings.

3 If *Pneumocystis carinii* pneumonia (PCP) is suspected, start treatment immediately (Table 46.4).

- Seek expert advice, as treatment regimens are developing rapidly.
- Steroid therapy should be given to patients with severe PCP (Table 46.5).

- Zidovudine (AZT) should be stopped while treating PCP.

Further management

This will depend on the diagnosis. Seek expert advice from a chest physician.

■ **Table 46.1** Care of HIV+ patient: safety precautions

- Cover all abrasions with a waterproof plaster
- Wear latex gloves and plastic apron when handling urine, faeces, drain fluid or blood
- Wear mask and visor or goggles for tracheobronchial suctioning
- Wear a single use, non-absorbent surgeon's gown for inserting central lines, intra-arterial lines or invasive procedures such as endoscopy

■ **Table 46.2** Urgent investigation of the breathless HIV+ patient

- Chest X-ray
- Arterial blood gases and pH
- Full blood count
- Blood culture (positive in most patients with *Mycobacterium avium-intracellulare* infection)
- Urea, sodium and potassium
- Sputum (if available) for Gram and Ziehl–Nielson stain and culture

Other investigations to discuss with a chest physician

- Examination of induced sputum
- Fibreoptic bronchoscopy (for bronchoalveolar lavage or transbronchial biopsy)

■ **Table 46.3** Diagnostic clues in the breathless HIV+ patient

Diagnosis	Clinical	Chest X-ray
Pneumocystis carinii pneumonia (PCP)	Dyspnoea (often slow onset) Dry cough Lungs clear or sparse basal crackles Fever	Perihilar haze common Lobar consolidation rare Pleural effusion rare
Mycobacterium avium intracellulare infection	Cough Dyspnoea Fever	Often normal
Bacterial pneumonia (p. 173)	Commoner in smokers Productive cough Focal signs Fever	Focal consolidation
Cytomegalovirus pneumonitis	Clinically indistinguishable from PCP (dual infection may occur)	Diffuse bilateral interstitial shadowing
Kaposi's sarcoma	No fever Dyspnoea More common in homosexual men and Africans than IV drug users May be associated with cutaneous Kaposi's sarcoma	Diffuse interstitial shadowing, more nodular than PCP May be unilateral and associated with hilar adenopathy Pleural effusion strongly suggestive

Neurological problems (Table 46.6)

With improved PCP prophylaxis, HIV+ patients are presenting more frequently with neurological problems.

Confusion with or without headache

• Consider HIV encephalopathy, cryptococcal meningitis, and toxoplasmosis.

■ **Table 46.4** Treatment of *Pneumocystis carinii* pneumonia

Antimicrobial therapy: cotrimoxazole or pentamidine

Cotrimoxazole
0.625 ml/kg 12-hourly IV
Dilute 1 : 25 in 5% dextrose or saline; give over 90 min.
If neutrophil count $< 1.5 \times 10^9$/l, give folinic acid 15 mg once daily PO and
   reduce dose to 75%
Causes haemolysis in glucose-6-phosphate dehydrogenase deficient patients
   (African/Mediterranean)

Pentamidine
4 mg/kg once daily IV
Make up to 250 ml with 5% dextrose: give over 1 hour with the patient lying
   flat
Watch for hyotension
Can cause renal impairment

**Steroid therapy: start immediately if severe PCP (see Table 46.5) or if
deteriorating on treatment**

Several different regimens are recommended. One commonly used in the
UK is:
● methylprednisolone 1 g/day IV for 3 days
If improved, stop; if not:
● methylprednisolone 500 mg/day IV for 2 more days, then
● prednisolone 60 mg/day PO reducing to 0 over 10 days

● Arrange urgent computed tomography (CT) scan (or magnetic
resonance imaging (MRI)).
● Perform lumbar puncture after CT if there is no contraindication.
Send **cerebrospinal fluid (CSF)** for: **cell count; protein concentration;
glucose** (fluoride tube); **Gram, Ziehl–Nielson and India ink stains;
serological tests for *Cryptococcus* and *Toxoplasma gondii*.**

Focal upper motor neuron signs

● Consider toxoplasmosis or lymphoma.
● Arrange urgent CT scan (or MRI if available).

■ **Table 46.5** Clinical grading of *Pneumocystis carinii* pneumonia

Feature	Mild	Moderate	Severe
Clinical	Increasing exertional dyspnoea	Dyspnoea on minimal exertion; fever	Dyspnoea at rest; cough; fever
Arterial oxygen tension breathing room air (kPa)	>11 (falls with exercise)	$8-11$	<8
Chest X-ray	Normal or minor perihilar shadowing	Diffuse interstitial shadowing	Extensive interstitial shadowing with or without diffuse alveolar shadowing (sparing costophrenic angles and apices)

Reference:
Miller RF, Mitchell D. *Thorax* 1992: 47; 305–14.

• Perform lumbar puncture after CT if there is no contraindication, and send CSF for investigation as above.
• If focal lesions are seen on CT, treat as toxoplasmosis. If there is no response, consider brain biopsy.

Impaired vision

• Suspect cytomegalovirus retinitis: fundoscopy shows characteristic infiltrates, similar in appearance to soft exudates.
• Seek an opthalmological opinion urgently.
• Treatment is with ganciclovir or foscarnet; zidovudine should be stopped during treatment.

■ Table 46.6 Neurological problems in HIV/AIDS

Diagnosis	Clinical features	CT scan	Tests	Treatment
Cryptococcal meningitis (pp. 209–10)	Insidious onset Confusional state Fever Headache Meningism rare	Normal	CSF may stain positive Cryptococcal antigen in blood and CSF	Fluconazole or amphotericin (avoid if liver function tests abnormal; nephrotoxic)
Toxoplasmosis	Confusional state Focal UMN signs	Single or frequently multiple space-occupying lesions	Serology positive (but common without active toxoplasmosis)	Pyrimethamine (folinic acid supplement needed) and sulphadiazine Stop zidovudine during treatment
Lymphoma	Insidious onset Confusional state Focal UMN signs	Multiple space-occupying lesions	Brain biopsy	Radiotherapy/chemotherapy

UMN, Upper motor neuron.

Appendix 1: spectrum of HIV infection

■ **Table 46.7** Spectrum of HIV infection

Group 1	Acute infection
Group 2	Asymptomatic infection
Group 3	Persistent generalized lymphadenopathy
Group 4	Other disease

Group 4 — Other disease

Constitutional disease (e.g. fever, weight loss, diarrhoea)*

Neurological disease (HIV encephalopathy, opportunistic infection, central nervous system lymphoma)

Secondary infectious diseases
- *Pneumocystis carinii* pneumonia
- *Cytomegalovirus* chorioretinitis, colitis, pneumonitis or adrenalitis
- *Candida albicans:* oral thrush*, oesophagitis
- *Mycobacterium avium-intracellulare* localized or disseminated infection
- *Mycobacterium tuberculosis* infection*
- *Cryptococcus neoformans:* meningitis or disseminated infection
- *Toxoplasma gondii:* encephalitis or intracerebral mass lesions
- *Herpes simplex* virus: severe mucocutaneous lesions, oesophagitis
- *Cryptosporidium* diarrhoea
- *Isospora belli* diarrhoea

Secondary neoplasms
- Kaposi's sarcoma (cutaneous and visceral)
- Lymphoma (brain, bone marrow, gut)

Other conditions (thrombocytopenia, non-specific interstitial pneumonitis)*

AIDS is diagnosed in an HIV+ patient with group 4 disease, except those marked*.

47 Septic arthritis

- Consider the diagnosis in any patient with **fever and joint swelling** (particularly if only one large joint is involved).
- Other causes of acute arthritis are listed in Table 47.1. Important points in the clinical assessment are given in Table 47.2.

Priorities

1 Aspirate the joint and send synovial fluid for: **cell count** (EDTA tube) (normal $< 180/mm^3$, most mononuclear); **Gram stain; culture**; and **microscopy under polarized light for crystals**. If you are not familiar with joint aspiration, seek the help of a rheumatologist or orthopaedic surgeon.

- Both crystal and septic arthritis give rise to a purulent effusion, although the white-cell count is usually higher in septic arthritis ($50\,000-200\,000/mm^3$).
- Blood-staining of the effusion is common in pseudogout but rare in sepsis.

2 Other investigations are given in Table 47.3.

Further management

Organisms on Gram stain of synovial fluid, or high probability of septic arthritis

- Start antibiotic therapy IV (Table 47.4). Intra-articular administration is not needed. The antibiotic regimen may need modification in the light of blood and synovial fluid culture results: discuss this with the microbiologist.
- **If septic arthritis is confirmed, seek expert advice** on further management of the joint from a rheumatologist or orthopaedic surgeon.

■ **Table 47.1** Causes of acute arthritis

Usually mono- or oligoarthritis

- Acute crystal arthritis: gout and pseudogout
- Non-gonococcal septic arthritis
- Haemarthrosis (in haemophilia)
- Osteoarthritis
- Trauma (causing internal derangement, haemarthrosis or fracture, or acute synovitis from penetrating injury)

Usually polyarthritis

- Gonococcal arthritis
- Reactive arthritis following gut or genital infection
- Rheumatic diseases, e.g. rheumatoid arthritis, SLE
- Viral infections, e.g. rubella, hepatitis A and B, infectious mononucleosis

SLE, Systemic lupus erythematosus.

■ **Table 47.2** Clinical assessment of the patient with acute arthritis

- **Arthritis or periarticular inflammation** (bursitis, tendinitis or cellulitis)? Painful limitation of movement of the joint suggests arthritis
- **Source of infection** (e.g. pneumonia, urinary tract infection, soft-tissue abscess)? Septic arthritis usually follows a bacteraemia
- **Risk factor for septic arthritis** (rheumatoid arthritis, prosthetic joint, IV drug abuse, immunocompromised)?
- **History of trauma?**
- **Recent diuretic therapy** (may precipitate gout)?
- **Sexual activity** – at risk of sexually transmitted disease?
- **Previous similar attack?** This supports the diagnosis of crystal or other non-infectious arthritis
- **Associated rash, diarrhoea, urethritis or uveitis?**

- Aspirate the joint daily until an effusion no longer reaccumulates.
- While the infection is resolving, the joint should be immobilized using a splint or cast.
- Physiotherapy should be started early.

■ Table 47.3 Investigation in suspected septic arthritis

- Joint aspiration
- X-ray joint to exclude osteomyelitis and for baseline
- Chest X-ray to exclude pneumonia
- Full blood count
- C-reactive protein and ESR
- Blood culture
- Urine microscopy and culture
- Swab of urethra, cervix and ano-rectum if gonococcal infection is possible (see Appendix 1)

ESR, Erythrocyte sedimentation rate.

■ Table 47.4 Initial antibiotic therapy for suspected septic arthritis

Organism on Gram stain	Antibiotic
Gram positive cocci	Flucloxacillin 1 g 6-hourly IV
Gram negative cocci	Benzylpenicillin 1.2 g 6-hourly IV
Gram negative rods	Gentamicin (dosage: p. 84) IV
None seen	
• Gonococcal infection likely	Benzylpenicillin
• Gonococcal infection unlikely	Benzylpenicillin plus Flucloxacillin

- Give non-steroidal anti-inflammatory drug (NSAID) for pain relief (e.g. indomethacin or diclofenac).
- In patients with gonococcal arthritis, sexual partners should be traced.

No organisms on Gram stain of synovial fluid and low probability of septic arthritis

- Consider the other causes of acute arthritis (see Table 47.1). Pseudogout is the commonest cause of acute mono- or oligoarthritis in the elderly.

- Hold off antibiotic therapy (pending the results of blood and synovial fluid culture for definite exclusion of infection).
- Treat with NSAID.
- If gout is confirmed (also check plasma urate) and fails to respond to NSAID, use colchicine. Allopurinol should not be started until the acute attack has completely resolved.

Appendix 1

■ **Table 47.4** Comparison of gonococcal and non-gonococcal septic arthritis

	Gonococcal	Non-gonococcal
At risk	• Sexually active	• Elderly • Rheumatoid arthritis • Prosthetic joint • IV drug abuse • Immunocompromised
Organisms	• N. gonorrhoeae	• Staphylococcus aureus (60%) • Gram-negative bacteria (18%) • Beta-haemolytic streptococci (15%) • Streptococcus pneumoniae (3%)
Joints involved	• Often polyarticular, esp. knee and wrist	• Usually monoarticular, esp. knee
Other signs	• Tenosynovitis • Rash	• Underlying illness • Source of bacteraemia
Gram stain of synovial fluid	• < 25% positive	• 50–75% positive
Culture of synovial fluid	• 25% positive	• 85–95% positive
Blood culture Genitourinary culture*	• < 10% positive • 80% positive	• 50% positive

* Swab of urethra, cervix and anorectum.

References:
Goldenberg DL, Reed JI. Bacterial arthritis. *N Engl J Med* 1985; 312: 764–71.
Baker DG, Schumacher HR Jr. Acute monoarthritis. *N Engl J Med* 1993; 329: 1013–20.

48 Anaphylactic shock

1 Suspect anaphylaxis if, **after an IV/IM injection, insect sting or exposure to a potential allergen**, the patient develops:
- **skin and mucosal urticaria, erythema and angioedema;**
- **wheeze and breathlessness;**
- **tachycardia and hypotension.**

2 Causes of anaphylactic reaction are given in Table 48.1.

Priorities

1 **If cardiac arrest appears imminent, give adrenaline 0.5–1 mg IV** (5–10 ml of 1 in 10 000 solution, 0.5–1 ml of 1 in 1000 solution). **If there is no IV access, give it IM or SC.**

2 **Give oxygen 100%. If there is respiratory distress, call an anaesthetist:** this may be due to **upper airways obstruction** from oedema of the larynx or epiglottis, and may require **endotracheal intubation or emergency tracheotomy.**

3 **Put in an IV cannula. If systolic BP is < 90 mmHg, give an IV infusion of colloid,** 500 ml over 15–30 min.

4 **Attach an ECG monitor** (as arrhythmias may occur with IV administration of adrenaline).

5 **If there is bronchospasm, give nebulized salbutamol** supplemented by **aminophylline IV** if required (p. 164).

6 **Give chlorpheniramine 10 mg IV over 1 min and hydrocortisone 300 mg IV.**

7 **If the patient remains hypotensive:**
- **continue IV colloid infusion** – put in a central venous line to guide the rate of infusion;
- **give further doses of adrenaline** 0.5–1 mg IV every 10 min or start an infusion (p. 374). If the patient has been taking a beta-blocker and is resistant to adrenaline, give **glucagon** (50 µg/kg by IV bolus followed by an infusion of 1–5 mg/hour) or **noradrenaline** (p. 374).

■ **Table 48.1** Causes of anaphylactic and anaphylactoid reaction*

Drugs
- Antibiotics, most commonly beta-lactam class
- Radiographic contrast media
- Parenteral iron
- Streptokinase
- Neuromuscular blocking agents
- Thiopentone
- Vitamin K

Blood products

Allergen extracts

Bee and wasp stings

* Anaphylactic and anaphylactoid reactions to drugs are clinically indistinguishable. Anaphylactoid reactions are due to direct triggering of the release of mediators by the drug itself and may therefore occur after the first dose.

Further management

1 Admit for 24 hours as relapses can occur.

2 Give hydrocortisone 300 mg 6-hourly IV for 2−4 doses and chlor-pheniramine 8 mg 8-hourly PO for 24−48 hours.

3 Inform the patient of the drug responsible for the reaction.

- A bracelet engraved with this information may be obtained from Medic-alert Foundation International, 12 Bridge Wharf, 156 Caledonian Road, London N1 9UU (tel. 0171-833 3034).

- If appropriate, adrenaline for self-injection in the event of further exposure to allergen may be obtained from International Medication Systems UK Ltd (Min-I-Jet adrenaline 1 : 1000 1 mg/1 ml with integral SC needle 25G, 0.25 inch). Adrenaline may also be administered by a metered-dose inhaler (Medihaler-Epi, 3M, 0.154 mg of adrenaline base per puff).

4 If anaphylaxis was due to a drug, report the reaction to the

Committee on Safety of Medicines (see the Adverse Reactions to Drugs section of the *British National Formulary*).

5 Specific allergen immunotherapy (desensitization) is indicated in the case of severe anaphylactic reaction to bee or wasp stings: seek expert advice from a clinical immunologist.

Minor anaphylactic reaction

Give chlorpheniramine 10 mg IV (repeated only if symptoms recur).

49 Sickle-cell crisis

1 The commonest complication of sickle-cell disease in adults is a vaso-occlusive crisis with infarction of bone marrow.

2 Suspect a vaso-occlusive crisis in any black, Arabic, Indian or Mediterranean patient with **acute pain in the spine, abdomen, chest or joints**. Most patients with sickle-cell disease will know their diagnosis.

3 **Make a working diagnosis from:**
- the sickle solubility test and blood film;
- the presence of a likely precipitant (infection, dehydration, strenuous exercise, exposure to cold and psychological stress);
- the exclusion of other causes where possible.

Priorities

1 **Relieve pain.**
- **If the pain is severe, give morphine by continuous SC or IV infusion:** give a loading dose of 10 mg SC (5 mg if < 50 kg), followed by an infusion of 150 µg/kg/hour, titrating the dose to time to breakthrough of pain. Monitor respiratory rate and oxygen saturation by pulse oximetry.
- Mild pain can be treated with a non-steroidal anti-inflammatory drug (NSAID).

2 Assess the patient for **evidence of infection, neurological or pulmonary involvement, and to exclude other causes of pain**. Investigations required urgently are given in Table 49.1.
- Adults with sickle-cell disease are effectively splenectomized and thus at particular risk of infection with capsulate bacteria: *Pneumococcus*, *Meningococcus* and *Haemophilus influenzae* type B.
- Fever may occur without infection (reflecting tissue necrosis).
- Antibiotic therapy should be started after taking blood for culture. If there is no clinical focus of infection, give amoxycillin.

3 **Indications for exchange transfusion** are given in Table 49.2.

■ **Table 49.1** Urgent investigation of suspected vaso-occlusive crisis of sickle-cell disease

- Steady-state haemoglobin and haemoglobin electrophoresis from clinic card if diagnosis established
- Full blood count, reticulocyte count and film*
- Sickle solubility test† (haemoglobin electrophoresis as soon as practicable)
- Blood culture
- Urine microscopy and culture
- Chest X-ray
- Oxygen saturation by pulse oximetry
- Arterial blood gases (if chest X-ray shadowing, or respiratory symptoms)

*Blood film in sickle cell disease (homozygous SS): normochromic normocytic anaemia; raised reticulocyte count; in adults, Howell–Jolly bodies (reflecting hyposplenism), usually sickle cells. Numerous target cells indicate haemoglobin SC.

†Sickle solubility test indicates the presence of haemoglobin S, and is therefore positive in both homozygotes (SS) and heterozygotes (AS – sickle-cell trait), and also double heterozygotes (S beta Thal, SC).

■ **Table 49.2** Indications for exchange transfusion in complications of sickle-cell disease

- Neurological involvement: stroke, transient ischaemic attack or fits
- Lung involvement ($Pa_{O_2} < 9$ kPa with FI_{O_2} 60%)
- Sequestration syndromes
- Priapism

Seek expert advice on the management of these patients from a haematologist.

4 Is there chest involvement – pleuritic chest pain with X-ray shadowing? This carries a relatively high mortality. It is impossible to distinguish vaso-occlusive infarction from pneumonia with certainty and you should assume that both coexist.

- Give oxygen 28–60% by mask and monitor oxygen saturation by pulse oximetry, aiming to maintain $Sa_{O_2} > 90\%$. Recheck arterial gases after 4 hours or if deterioration occurs. Ventilation and

exchange transfusion are needed if Pa_{O_2} cannot be maintained above 9 kPa (70 mmHg) with 60% oxygen by mask.
- Start antibiotic therapy (p. 176).

Further management

1 **Ensure a fluid intake of 3 l/m^2 daily** (in most cases, start with an IV infusion) and keep the patient warm.
2 **Check haemoglobin daily:** discuss management with a haematologist if the haemoglobin is falling or reticulocytes are absent (which may indicate an aplastic or sequestration crisis).

Problems

Vaso-occlusive crisis or acute abdomen?

- There is no clear distinction and the patient should be assessed jointly with the surgical team.
- It is often reasonable to delay surgery longer than usual and to proceed if deterioration occurs despite treatment directed at vaso-occlusive crisis.

Sickle crises causing increased anaemia

These are much less common than vaso-occlusive crises:
- sequestration crisis (in the sinuses of the enlarged spleen in children);
- aplastic crisis (reduced marrow erythropoiesis, e.g. after parvovirus infection);
- haemolytic crisis (following infections).

The clue is the rapid fall in haemoglobin. These crises must be recognized early because transfusion can be life-saving. Seek expert advice from a haematologist.

50 Fever on return from abroad

- **Exclude malaria or typhoid in any febrile illness within 2 months of return from an endemic area** (most of Africa, Asia, Central and South America: for further information contact a specialist centre (Appendix 2)).
- Chemoprophylaxis against malaria does not ensure full protection and may prolong the incubation period.
- **The clinical features of malaria are non-specific: diagnosis requires examination of a blood film for parasites.**

Priorities

1 Admit to a single room and nurse with standard isolation technique until the diagnosis is established.
2 In patients who have travelled to rural west Africa within the previous 3 weeks, a viral haemorrhagic fever must be considered, particularly if pharyngitis is a prominent symptom: seek expert advice from an infectious-diseases physician on management (before blood samples are taken).
3 Investigations needed urgently are given in Table 50.2.

Further management

This depends upon associated features:

Septic shock

- Antimicrobial therapy must cover **falciparum malaria** (Appendix 1) and **typhoid** (Table 50.3) in patients who have travelled to endemic regions.
- Patients with **falciparum malaria** must also receive antibiotics to

■ **Table 50.1** Infectious diseases that may be acquired abroad

	Incubation periods	
Infection	**Usual**	**Range**
Malaria		
Plasmodium falciparum	12 days	8–25 days
Plasmodium vivax	15 days	8–27 days
Plasmodium malariae	28 days	15–30 days
Plasmodium ovale	15 days	9–17 days
Typhoid	10–14 days	7–21 days
Leptospirosis	10 days	7–13 days
Legionella pneumophila	10 days	2–26 days
Hepatitis A	4 weeks	2–6 weeks
Hepatitis B	12 weeks	6 weeks to 6 months

■ **Table 50.2** Urgent investigation of fever on return from abroad

- **Full blood count** (neutropenia is seen in both malaria and typhoid; a low platelet count is common in falciparum malaria)
- **Blood film for malarial parasites** if travel to or through an endemic area; the intensity of the parasitaemia is variable and if the diagnosis is suspected but the film is negative, repeat blood films every 8 hours for 2–3 days
- **Urea, sodium and potassium**
- **Blood glucose**
- **Blood culture** (positive in 70–90% of patients in the first week of typhoid)
- **Throat swab**
- **Urine** stick test, microscopy and culture
- **Stool** microscopy and culture
- **Chest X-ray**
- **Lumbar puncture** if neck stiffness present

For later analysis

- **Liver function tests**
- **Serology** as appropriate (e.g. for suspected viral hepatitis, *Legionella pneumonia*, typhoid, amoebic liver abscess, leptospirosis)

■ **Table 50.3** Typhoid

Clinical features

• Insidious onset with headache, malaise, anorexia and fever; dry cough common
• Initial constipation followed later by diarrhoea
• Abdominal pain, distension and tenderness
• Liver and spleen often palpable after first week
• Erythematous macular rash (rose spots) on upper abdomen and anterior chest may occur during second week

Antibiotic therapy (give for 14 days)

Severely ill	• Ciprofloxacin 200 mg 12-hourly IV; or • Chloramphenicol 500 mg 4-hourly IV, reducing to 500 mg 6-hourly PO when afebrile
Others	• Ciprofloxacin 500–750 mg 12-hourly PO

cover **Gram-negative infection** (as mixed infections may occur).
• See Chapter 10 for general management.

Chest X-ray shadowing

Consider **pulmonary tuberculosis** and *Legionella* **pneumonia** (p. 178) in addition to the common causes of pneumonia.

Meningism

• Perform a lumbar puncture. If the cerebrospinal fluid (CSF) shows no organisms but a high lymphocyte count, consider **tuberculous meningitis** (p. 209), **leptospirosis**, or **brucellosis**.
• If there are other features suggesting **leptospirosis** (haemorrhagic rash, conjunctivitis, renal failure, jaundice) give benzylpenicillin 600 mg 4-hourly IV for 7 days. Alternative antibiotics are erythromycin or tetracycline.

Jaundice

- Always consider **falciparum malaria**.
- Other causes are **hepatitis A and B** (but with these infections patients are afebrile when jaundice appears), **leptospirosis**, **cytomegalovirus** and **Epstein–Barr virus infection**.

Appendix 1: treatment of malaria

Chemotherapy

If the infective species is not known, or if the infection is mixed, initial treatment should be with quinine, mefloquine or halofantrine as for falciparum malaria.

Falciparum malaria

Patient seriously ill or unable to take tablets
Quinine should be given by IV infusion.
- **Loading dose:** 20 mg/kg (up to a maximum of 1.4 g) of quinine salt given over 4 hours by IV infusion (omit if quinine or mefloquin given within the previous 24 hours), followed after 8–12 hours by:
- **Maintenance dose:** 10 mg/kg (up to a maximum of 700 mg) of quinine salt given over 4 hours by IV infusion 8–12-hourly, until the patient can swallow tablets to complete the 7 day course. Reduce the maintenance dose to 5–7 mg/kg of quinine salt if IV treatment is needed for more than 48 hours.

Patient is not seriously ill and can swallow tablets
Treat with one of the three regimens listed below.
- **Quinine** 600 mg of quinine salt 8-hourly PO for 7 days, followed by either a single dose of three tablets of **Fansidar** (each tablet contains pyrimethamine 25 mg and sulfadoxine 500 mg), or (if Fansidar-resistant) **tetracycline** 250 mg 6-hourly PO for 7 days when renal function has returned to normal.

- **Mefloquine** 20 mg/kg (up to a maximum of 1.5 g) as a single dose or preferably two divided doses 6–8 hours apart PO.
- **Halofantrine** 1.5 g of halofantrine hydrochloride divided into three doses of 500 mg given 6-hourly PO. This course should be repeated after 1 week.

It is not necessary to give Fansidar or tetracycline after treatment with mefloquine or halofantrine.

Points in the management of severe falciparum malaria
1 Admit to the intensive-therapy unit.
2 Start chemotherapy with quinine IV (see above) as soon as possible.
3 Obtain expert advice on management (Appendix 2).
4 Patients with reduced conscious level may have **cerebral malaria** (Table 50.4), but CSF should be examined to exclude coexistent bacterial meningitis. If there are focal signs or papilloedema, computed tomography must be done before lumbar puncture, to exclude a mass lesion. In this case, take blood cultures and start antibacterial therapy (Table 30.3, p. 205) first.

Specific problems that may be encountered
1 Hypotension.
- Give colloid (or blood if packed cell volume $< 20\%$, haemoglobin < 7 g/dl) to maintain central venous pressure (CVP) at $+5$ cm water (avoid higher levels because of the risk of pulmonary oedema).
- Start antibiotic therapy for Gram-negative sepsis after taking blood cultures (p. 80).
- Start inotrope/vasopressor agents if needed (p. 40).

2 Hypoglycaemia.
- Blood glucose should be checked 4-hourly, or if conscious level deteriorates or fits occur.
- If blood glucose is < 3.5 mmol/l, give 50 ml of 50% dextrose IV and start an IV infusion of 10% dextrose (initially 1 l 12-hourly) via a large peripheral or central vein.

3 Fits.
- Recheck blood glucose.
- Manage along standard lines (p. 218).

■ **Table 50.4** Cerebral malaria: clinical features

- **Reduced conscious level**
- **Focal or generalized fits** common
- **Abnormal neurological signs** may be present (including opisthotonos, extensor posturing of decorticate or decerebrate pattern, sustained posturing of limbs, conjugate deviation of the eyes, nystagmus, dysconjugate eye movements, bruxism, extensor plantar responses, generalized flaccidity)
- **Retinal haemorrhages** common (papilloedema may be present but is unusual)
- **Abnormal patterns of breathing** common (including irregular periods of apnoea and hyperventilation)

Reference:
Molyneux M, Fox R. Diagnosis and treatment of malaria in Britain. *BMJ* 1993; 306: 1175–80.

4 Pulmonary oedema.
- May occur from excessive IV fluid or acute respiratory distress syndrome (ARDS) (p. 140).
- Mechanical ventilation may be needed.

Benign malarias

Plasmodium vivax and *ovale* malaria
Give 600 mg of **chloroquine** base PO, followed by a single dose of 300 mg after 6–8 hours, followed by 300 mg daily 2 days. Then give **primaquine** 15 mg daily PO for 14–21 days to eradicate the exo-erythrocytic cycle. **Check for glucose-6-phosphate dehydrogenase (G6PD) deficiency first** as the drug can cause haemolysis in patients who are deficient in the enzyme: if G6PD-deficient, give 30 mg once weekly for 8 weeks.

Plasmodium malariae malaria
Chloroquine alone is sufficient, following the above regimen.

Appendix 2: UK reference centres for advice on malaria treatment

London

Hospital for Tropical Diseases
4 St Pancras Way
London NW1 0PE
Telephone: 0171 3874411

Lister Unit
Northwick Park Hospital
Harrow
Middlesex
Telephone: 0181 8692831/2

Birmingham

Department of Communicable and Tropical Diseases
East Birmingham Hospital
Bordesley Green East
Birmingham B9 5ST
Telephone: 0121 7724311

Liverpool

School of Tropical Medicine
Pembroke Place
Liverpool L3 5QA
Telephone: 0151 9246852

Oxford

Centre for Tropical Medicine
John Radcliffe Hospital

Headington
Oxford OX3 9DU
Telephone: 01865 741166

Glasgow

Communicable Diseases (Scotland) Unit
Ruchill Hospital
Glasgow
G20 9NB
Telephone: 0141 9467120

Section 3
Procedures

51 Central vein cannulation

Indications

1 Measurement of central venous pressure (CVP) (Table 51.1 and Fig. 51.1):
- transfusion of large volumes of fluid required;
- fluid challenge in patients with oliguria or hypotension;
- to exclude hypovolaemia when the clinical evidence is equivocal.

2 Insertion of a pulmonary artery (Swan–Ganz) catheter or temporary pacing wire.

3 Administration of some drugs (e.g. dopamine) and IV feeding solutions.

4 No suitable peripheral veins for IV infusion.

NB: central vein cannulation has many potential complications (Table 51.2): give careful consideration to the need for the procedure and the choice of vein.

■ **Table 51.1** Interpreting the central venous pressure

The CVP reflects the interaction between blood volume, systemic venous tone, right ventricular function and intrathoracic/pericardial pressure

Causes of a high CVP

- Fluid overload, e.g. renal failure, overtransfusion
- Right ventricular failure, e.g. right ventricular infarction, major pulmonary embolism
- Tension pneumothorax
- Cardiac tamponade

Causes of a low CVP

- Hypovolaemia, e.g. diabetic hyperglycaemic states
- Vasodilatation, e.g. sepsis, poisoning

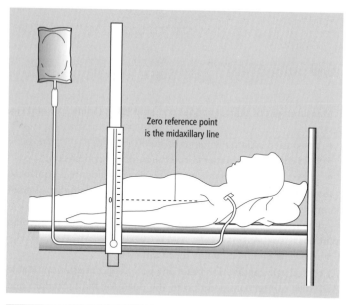

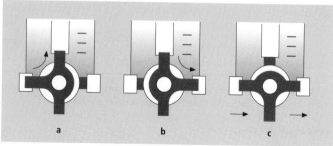

Fig. 51.1 Method of measuring CVP. CVP line with position of three-way tap for: **a**, priming the manometer; **b**, measuring CVP; **c**, fluid infusion. From Davidson TI. *Fluid balance*. Oxford: Blackwell Scientific Publications, 1987; 38.

■ **Table 51.2** Complications of central vein cannulation

During placement

- Arterial puncture or laceration
- Pneumothorax (via internal jugular or subclavian vein) or tension pneumothorax
- Haemothorax
- Cardiac tamponade (can be caused by central venous line introduced by any route, if its tip lies below the pericardial reflection and it perforates the vessel wall; least likely via internal jugular vein)
- Injury to adjacent nerves
- Air embolism

After placement

- Infection: local infection and/or bacteraemia
- Venous thrombosis

■ **Table 51.3** Choice of route for central vein cannulation

Vein	Comment
Internal jugular	Indicated in preference to subclavian vein if there is bleeding tendency or respiratory disease
Subclavian	Overall complication rate is higher than via internal jugular vein
Femoral	Safe route if rapid access required. Use for placing pulmonary artery catheter or pacing wire if access via internal jugular or subclavian veins is not possible. Drawbacks are increased risk of infection and venous thrombosis
Antecubital fossa vein	Use if thrombolytic therapy has been given. Often difficult to place pulmonary artery catheter or pacing wire via this route

Choice of vein (Table 51.3)

The right internal jugular and the right subclavian are the two most commonly used veins. The right internal jugular vein is preferable to the left as it is contralateral to the thoracic duct and the circulation of the dominant hemisphere. Cannulation of the internal jugular vein is generally associated with fewer complications and is the preferred approach in patients with:

• **bleeding tendency** – platelet count $< 100 \times 10^{12}/l$ or prothrombin time $> 1.5 \times$ control (because of the risk of uncontrollable bleeding from inadvertent arterial puncture);

• **respiratory disease** (because of the risk of pneumothorax precipitating respiratory failure).

Technique

Positioning the patient (for internal jugular or subclavian vein puncture)

• Remove the pillow and position the patient with head-down tilt of the bed if possible (to fill out the vein and reduce the risk of air embolism in hypovolaemic patients).

• Turn the patient's head away from the side you are going to puncture.

Venepuncture

Internal jugular vein puncture – high approach avoiding the risk of pneumothorax (Fig. 51.2)

1 Locate the right carotid artery. The internal jugular vein is superficial, lateral and parallel to the artery.

2 Prepare and drape the skin.

3 Infiltrate the skin and subcutaneous tissues over the anterior edge of the sternocleidomastoid muscle at the level of the thyroid cartilage with 5 ml of lignocaine 1%.

4 Nick the skin over the vein with a small scalpel blade.

5 Identify the line of the carotid artery with your left hand. Insert the needle just lateral to this at an angle of 45° to the skin, aiming for the right nipple in men, or the right anterior superior iliac spine in women

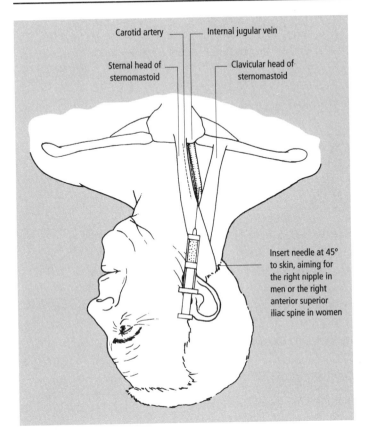

Carotid artery

Internal jugular vein

Sternal head of sternomastoid

Clavicular head of sternomastoid

Insert needle at 45° to skin, aiming for the right nipple in men or the right anterior superior iliac spine in women

Fig. 51.2 Right internal jugular vein puncture – high approach.

(see Fig. 51.2). A small gauge needle (e.g. 23G blue) can be used first to locate the vein. Advance slowly whilst aspirating for blood. The vein lies superficially so do not advance more than a few centimetres.

6 If you do not hit the vein, slowly withdraw the needle to just under the skin, again aspirating for blood (as you may have inadvertently transfixed the vein). Advance again, aiming slightly more medially.

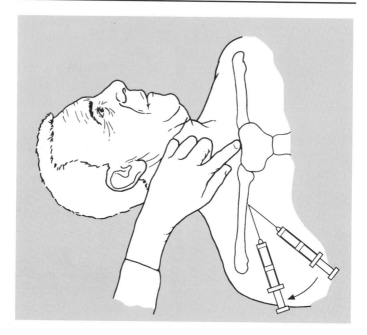

Fig. 51.3 Right subclavian vein puncture – infraclavicular approach.

Right subclavian vein puncture—infraclavicular
approach (Fig. 51.3)

1 Define the suprasternal notch, the sternoclavicular joint and the acromioclavicular joint.

2 Prepare and drape the skin.

3 Infiltrate the skin and subcutaneous tissues with 5–10 ml of lignocaine 1%, starting from a point one finger's breadth below the junction of the medial one-third and lateral two-thirds of the clavicle. Infiltrate up to and just below the clavicle.

4 Nick the skin with a small scalpel blade.

5 Advance the needle along the same track until it touches the clavicle. Move the tip stepwise down the clavicle until it is lying just below it. Then swing the needle round so that it is now pointing at the suprasternal notch (see Fig. 51.3). Slowly advance the needle whilst aspirating for blood. Make a conscious effort to keep the track of the needle parallel to the bed (to avoid puncturing the subclavian artery or pleura).

6 If the vein is not found, withdraw slowly whilst aspirating. Flush the needle to make sure it is not blocked. Try again, aiming slightly more cranially.

Right femoral vein puncture (Fig. 51.4)

1 Place the patient in a supine position. The leg should be slightly abducted and externally rotated. Identify the femoral artery below the inguinal ligament: the femoral vein lies medially.

2 If time allows, shave the groin. Prepare and drape the skin.

3 Infiltrate the skin and subcutaneous tissues with 5–10 ml of lignocaine 1%.

4 Nick the skin with a small scalpel blade.

5 Place two fingers of your left hand on the femoral artery to define its position. Holding the syringe in your right hand, place the tip of the needle at the entry site on the skin. Move the syringe slightly laterally, and advance the needle at an angle of around 30° to the skin whilst aspirating for blood (see Fig. 51.4). The vein is usually reached 2–4 cm from the skin surface.

6 If the vein is not found, withdraw slowly whilst aspirating. Flush the needle to make sure it is not blocked. Try again, aiming slightly to the left or right of your initial pass.

Placement of the cannula using a guidewire-through-needle technique (Seldinger technique)

1 Once you have punctured the vein, check that you can aspirate blood easily.

2 Remove the syringe, capping the needle to prevent entry of air.

3 Pass the flexible end of the guidewire down the needle. If there is any resistance to the passage of the wire, withdraw it and check you are still in the vein by aspirating blood. Change the angle of the needle or rotate the bevel. If there is still resistance, but you are confident the needle is in the vein, try a new wire with a flexible J-shaped end.

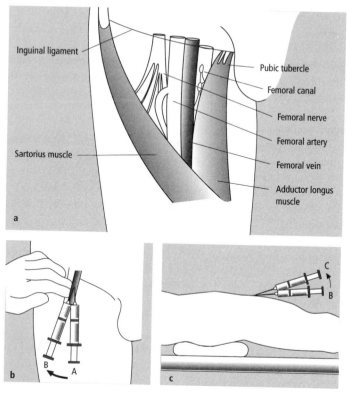

Fig. 51.4 Right femoral vein puncture: **a**, anatomy of the femoral vein; **b**, and **c**, technique. From Rosen M, *et al. Handbook of Percutaneous Central Venous Catheterisation.* 2nd edn. London: WB Saunders, 1993.

4 When half the length of the wire is in the vein, remove the needle. Place the cannula and dilator over the wire and advance it into position.

- A cannula inserted via the subclavian vein sometimes passes into the internal jugular vein rather than the superior vena cava. This can be checked for by aspirating 5 ml of blood and then injecting it swiftly whilst a colleague listens with the diaphragm of a stethoscope over the ipsilateral internal jugular vein. A bruit signifies misplacement.

5 Attach the infusion set.

6 Fix the cannula to the skin with a suture or a transparent adhesive dressing.

7 A chest X-ray should be taken to confirm correct positioning of the cannula and absence of pneumothorax.

Troubleshooting

1 Arterial puncture. If you inadvertently puncture the carotid artery, apply pressure for 5 min and then reattempt venepuncture.

2 Pneumothorax. If the patient is being mechanically ventilated, this may become a tension pneumothorax and you must insert a chest drain even if it is small (p. 348). For management of pneumothorax in patients who are not ventilated see p. 179.

3 Misplacement of a cannula inserted via the subclavian vein in the internal jugular vein. The cannula must be repositioned. Infusion of hypertonic solutions into the internal jugular vein may cause venous thrombosis.

4 Frequent ventricular extrasystoles or ventricular tachycardia may indicate that the tip of the cannula is lying against the tricuspid valve. Withdraw it a few centimetres.

5 Infection of the cannula. *Staphylococcus aureus* and *epidermidis* are the commonest pathogens, but infection with Gram-negative rods and fungi may occur in immunocompromised patients.

• **Obviously infected line** (tenderness, erythema and purulent discharge at the skin exit site): **(a)** the cannula must be removed and the tip sent for culture; **(b)** if the patient is febrile, take blood cultures and start antibiotic therapy. Give flucloxacillin (cefuroxime if penicillin allergic) plus gentamicin. If methicillin-resistant *S. aureus* infection is possible, give vancomycin plus gentamicin. If an organism is isolated, change therapy as appropriate. For *S. aureus* infection, continue IV antibiotic therapy for 2 weeks.

• **Possibly infected line** (fever or other systemic signs of sepsis, but no signs at the skin exit site): **(a)** take blood cultures from both a peripheral vein and via the cannula; **(b)** the decision to remove the cannula before culture results are back depends on the likelihood of it being infected — how long has the cannula been in and is there another source of infection? **(c)** if both blood cultures grow the same organism, the cannula must be removed and antibiotic therapy given.

52 Pulmonary artery catheterization

Indications

1 **Pulmonary oedema:**
   • to titrate further therapy after initial management (p. 136);
   • to differentiate acute respiratory distress syndrome (ARDS) from cardiogenic pulmonary oedema (p. 140).

2 **Hypotension** despite central venous pressure (CVP) of 10 cm water or more (i.e. not due to hypovolaemia).

3 **Suspected ventricular septal rupture** after myocardial infarction (p. 113) if echocardiography is not available.

NB: **Pulmonary artery catheterization is diagnostic not therapeutic. Make sure that the patient is adequately resuscitated and receives appropriate treatment during the procedure.**

Technique

Preparation

1 Set up the equipment (Fig. 52.1).

2 The pressure transducer must be zeroed and calibrated. The reference point for zero is usually taken at the fourth intercostal space in the midaxillary line, with the patient supine.

3 Connect the patient to the ECG monitor and put in a peripheral venous cannula.

4 Prepare the skin and apply drapes as for temporary cardiac pacing.

5 Check that the catheter can pass down the cannula, and check the balloon by inflating it with air (usually 1.5 ml). Leave the syringe attached.

6 Attach the manometer line to the channel of the distal (pulmonary artery) lumen and flush the dead space. If the catheter also has a proximal (right atrial) lumen, flush this channel with heparinized saline and leave the syringe attached.

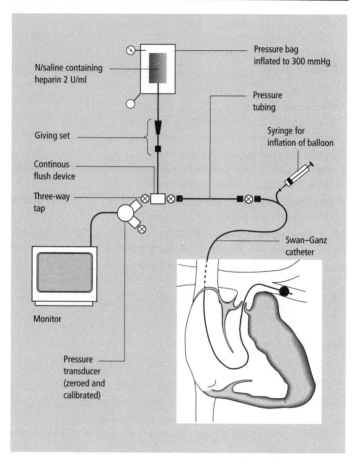

N/saline containing
heparin 2 U/ml

Pressure bag
inflated to 300 mmHg

Pressure
tubing

Giving set

Syringe for
inflation of balloon

Continous
flush device

Three-way
tap

Swan–Ganz
catheter

Monitor

Pressure
transducer
(zeroed and
calibrated)

Fig. 52.1 Diagram showing the set-up of equipment for pulmonary artery catheterization. When the balloon is inflated, flow around the tip of the catheter ceases. The measured pressure is transmitted back from the pulmonary veins (as these are valveless) and gives an estimate of left atrial and left ventricular end-diastolic pressure.

Cannulating a central vein

See Chapter 51.

Placement of the catheter

1 Insert the catheter for about 10 cm and inflate the balloon fully. Advance it guided by X-ray screening, or the pressure waveform (Fig. 52.2) and the distance inserted (Table 52.1). Do not advance more than 10–15 cm unless the waveform changes because of the risk of knotting.

- Always deflate the balloon before withdrawing the catheter to prevent it tearing the tricuspid or pulmonary valves.
- Ventricular extrasystoles and non-sustained ventricular tachycardia are common during manipulation of the catheter through the right heart and do not need treatment.
- Passage across the tricuspid valve can sometimes be helped by the patient taking a deep inspiration.

2 When the waveform changes from pulmonary artery to wedge, deflate the balloon. The trace should promptly change back to pulmonary artery.

■ **Table 52.1** Expected distance of catheter tip from point of insertion via right internal jugular vein in the adult

Location	Distance (cm)
Right atrium	10–15
Right ventricle	25–35
Pulmonary artery	35–40
Pulmonary artery wedge	40–50

Measuring the wedge pressure

Move the catheter to find a position where the wedge pressure is reliably obtained with the balloon fully or near-fully inflated. The

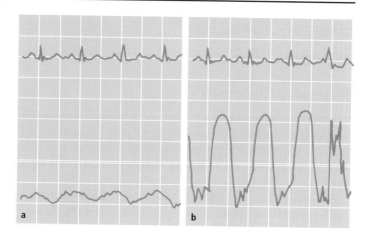

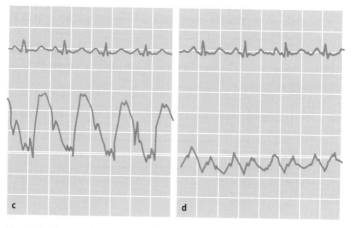

Fig. 52.2 Diagram showing the typical pressure waveforms on insertion of a Swan–Ganz catheter: **a**, right atrium; **b**, right ventricle; **c**, pulmonary artery; **d**, wedge position. See Appendix 1 for normal values.

■ **Table 52.2** Criteria of a satisfactory wedge position

1 The mean wedge pressure:
  • is lower than or equal to the PA diastolic pressure
  • is lower than the mean PA pressure
2 The waveform is characteristic of the left atrial waveform (see Fig. 52.3)
3 The wedge waveform promptly:
  • disappears on deflation of the balloon
  • reappears on reinflation
4 The balloon has to be inflated to its maximum volume (or close to this) to obtain the wedge pressure

PA, Pulmonary artery.

volume needed should be noted. If this is less than 1.3 ml, the catheter tip is too peripheral: withdraw it a little.
• Criteria of a satisfactory wedge position are given in Table 52.2.
• The wedge pressure fluctuates with respiration and should be measured at end-expiration when pleural pressure is around zero. Large swings in pleural pressure occur in patients with severe airways obstruction which can make interpretation of the wedge pressure trace difficult or impossible.
• Avoid keeping the balloon inflated in the wedge position for more than 15 s (to minimize the risk of pulmonary artery rupture).

Aftercare

• Obtain a chest X-ray to check the position of the catheter.
• Perform hourly fast flushes to prevent thrombus formation on the tip of the catheter.
• Remove the catheter within 72 hours to reduce the risk of infection. If needed, a new catheter can be put in, preferably at a different site.
• If infection related to the catheter is suspected: see p. 321.

Troubleshooting

The catheter will not enter the pulmonary artery

This can be a problem in patients with low cardiac output, tricuspid regurgitation or a dilated right heart.

If you cannot advance the catheter despite screening, use either a guidewire or stylet to stiffen it. Disconnect the catheter from the manometer line and pass a guidewire down the distal channel.

Damping of the pressure trace

This may be due to:
- kinking of the catheter or manometer line;
- air bubbles in the system;
- thrombus partially occluding the lumen of the catheter; several fast flushes should clear this.

Problems with measuring the wedge pressure

No change in waveform when you inflate the balloon
- If there is no resistance to inflation, suspect balloon rupture.
- If there is normal resistance, the catheter has slipped back. If the catheter outside the skin has not been kept sterile with a sheath, a new catheter should be inserted.

Ramp increase in pressure when you inflate the balloon
- This indicates that the balloon has inflated eccentrically with occlusion of the tip ('overwedging'). The ramp increase in pressure reflects the continuous flush infusion.
- Deflate the balloon and reinflate it until a satisfactory trace is obtained.

Tachypnoeic patient
- End-expiration is brief in a patient with rapid respiration and as the

monitor averages values obtained over several seconds, the digital display of the wedge pressure is misleading.
• The solution is to print out the pressure trace, marking end-expiration (most chart recorders will have an event marker) and measure the pressure from this.

Spontaneous wedging
• This indicates that the catheter is positioned too peripherally. Some migration peripherally commonly occurs after insertion as the catheter warms and becomes more flexible.
• Pull the catheter back until you find a position at which the balloon has to be fully or near-fully inflated to give a wedge pressure.

Special considerations

Suspected ventricular septal rupture
• Prepare four heparinized 2 ml syringes ready for sampling, with blind hubs and ice if the samples have to be transported to the laboratory.
• Take samples in the right atrium, right ventricle and pulmonary artery and from a systemic artery.
• A step-up in oxygen saturation of $> 10\%$ between right atrium and right ventricle indicates a left to right shunt at ventricular level.
• The size of the shunt is given by the ratio of pulmonary to systemic flow $(Q_P : Q_s)$, calculated as follows:

$$Q_P : Q_s = \frac{(Art - RA)}{(Art - PA)}$$

where Art is systemic arterial oxygen saturation (S_{O_2}), RA is right atrial S_{O_2} and PA is pulmonary arterial S_{O_2}.

Left bundle branch block
• Complete heart block is a rare and usually transient complication because the catheter may induce additional right bundle block as it passes through the right heart.
• Put in the catheter under screening, with a temporary pacing wire to hand in case this is needed.

Appendix 1

■ **Table 52.3** Pressure measurements: normal values

Site*	Pressure (mmHg)	
Central vein or right atrium	Mean	0−8
Right ventricle	Systolic	15−30
	Diastolic	0−8
Pulmonary artery (PA)	Systolic	15−30
	Diastolic†	3−12
	Mean	9−16
PA wedge pressure‡	Mean	1−10

* The **reference point for zero** is taken at the **fourth intercostal space in the midaxillary line** (the level of the tricuspid valve), with the patient lying flat.
† Pressures in the low-resistance pulmonary circulation normally equilibrate at end-diastole, and so the pulmonary artery diastolic pressure can substitute for the wedge pressure, providing: **(a)** the heart rate is less than 120/min; and **(b)** pulmonary hypertension is not present (PA systolic < 30 mmHg, PA mean < 20 mmHg).
‡ PA wedge pressure is measured at end-expiration, when pleural pressure is around zero and the intravascular pressure is closest to the physiologically relevant transmural pressure.

Appendix 2

■ Table 52.4 Derived variables

Variable	Formula	Normal range	Units
Body surface area	$\sqrt{\text{Height (inches)} \times \text{Weight (lb)}/3131}$; or $\sqrt{\text{Height (cm)} \times \text{Weight (kg)}/3600}$	—	m^2
Cardiac index	$CI = CO/BSA$	2.5–4.2	$l/min/m^2$
Systemic vascular resistance	$[MAP - RAP/CO \times 80]$	770–1500	$dyne.s/cm^5$
Pulmonary vascular resistance	$[MPAP - MPAWP/CO \times 80]$	25–125	$dyne.s/cm^5$
Arterial oxygen transport (Do_2)	$[0.134 \times CO \times Hba \times Sao_2]$	950–1300	ml/min
Systemic oxygen consumption (Vo_2)	$[0.134 \times CO \times (Hba \times Sao_2 - Hbv \times Svo_2)]$	180–320	ml/min
Alveolar–arterial oxygen gradient ($A - aDo_2$)	$Fio_2 \times 94.8 - (Pao_2 + Paco_2)$	< 3	kPa

BSA, Body surface area; CI, cardiac index; CO, cardiac output (l/min); Fio_2, fractional concentration of oxygen in inspired gas; Hba, haemoglobin concentration of arterial blood (g/dl); Hbv, haemoglobin concentration of venous blood (g/dl); MAP, mean systemic arterial pressure; MPAWP, mean pulmonary artery wedge pressure; MRAP, mean right atrial pressure; Sao_2, oxygen saturation of systemic arterial blood (%); Svo_2, oxygen saturation of mixed venous blood (%).

References:

Barry WH, Grossman W. Range of normal resting hemodynamic values. In: Braunwald E, ed. *Heart Disease: A Textbook of Cardiovascular Medicine*. 2nd edn. Philadelphia: WB Saunders, 1984.

Mosteller RD. Simplified calculation of body surface area. *N Engl J Med* 1987; 317: 1098.

53 Temporary cardiac pacing

Indications

These are given in Table 53.1.

■ **Table 53.1** Indications for temporary pacing

Acute myocardial infarction

- Asystole
- Complete heart block
- Right bundle branch block with new left anterior hemiblock or left posterior hemiblock
- New left bundle branch block
- Mobitz type II second-degree AV block
- Mobitz type I second-degree AV block with hypotension not responsive to atropine
- Sinus bradycardia with hypotension or recurrent sinus pauses not responsive to atropine
- Atrial or ventricular overdrive pacing for recurrent ventricular tachycardia

Unrelated to myocardial infarction

- Sinus or junctional bradycardia associated with haemodynamic compromise and unresponsive to atropine
- Second-degree AV block or sinus arrest if associated with syncope or presyncope
- Complete heart block with syncope or presyncope
- Atrial or ventricular overdrive pacing for recurrent ventricular tachycardia

Preoperative

- Sinus node disease/second-degree Mobitz type I (Wenckebach) AV block/bundle branch block (including bifascicular block) only if history of syncope or presyncope
- Second-degree Mobitz type II AV block
- Complete heart block

AV, Atrioventricular.

Technique

Preparation

1 Check the screening equipment and make sure a defibrillator and other resuscitation equipment is to hand.

2 Connect an ECG monitor and put in a peripheral venous cannula. Make sure the ECG leads are off the chest (so they are not confused with the pacing wire when screening).

3 Put on mask, gown and gloves. Prepare the skin and apply drapes to a wide area. If it is likely that permanent pacing will be needed, use the right side in right-handed patients.

4 Check that the wire will pass down the cannula. Temporary pacing wires are usually 5 or 6 French and require a cannula one size larger.

Cannulating a central vein

See Chapter 51.

• The wire is usually easier to manipulate via the right internal jugular vein, but may be fixed more comfortably via the right sub-clavian vein.

• The femoral vein can be used if access via the internal jugular or subclavian veins is not possible.

Placement of the wire (Figs 53.1 and 53.2)

1 Advance the wire into the right atrium and direct it towards the apex of the right ventricle (just medial to the lateral border of the cardiac silhouette): it may cross the tricuspid valve easily.

2 If you have difficulty, form a loop of wire in the right atrium. With slight rotation and advancement of the wire, the loop should prolapse across the tricuspid valve.

3 Manipulate the wire so that the tip curves downwards at the apex of the right ventricle and lies in a gentle S-shape within the right

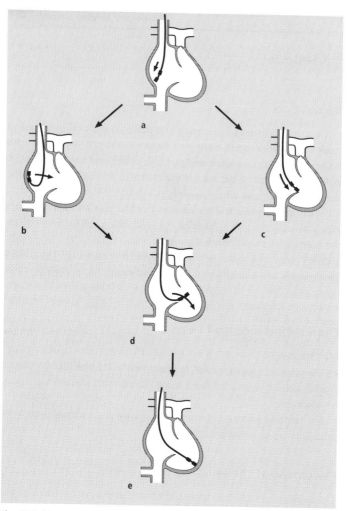

Fig. 53.1 Placement of a ventricular pacing wire from the superior vena cava (via internal jugular or subclavian veins): **a**, catheter advanced to the low right atrium; **b**, further advancement produces a loop or bend in the distal catheter, which is then rotated medially; **c**, alternatively, catheter in low-right atrium deflects off tricuspid annulus directly into the right ventricle; **d**, superior orientation of the catheter tip in the ventricle requires clockwise torque during advancement to avoid the interventricular septum; **e**, final catheter position in the right apex. Catheter position in b is suitable for atrial pacing. From Ellenbogen KA, ed. *Cardiac Pacing*. Boston: Blackwell Scientific Publications, 1992; 178–9.

atrium and ventricle (Fig. 53.3). Displacement of the wire may occur if there is too much or not enough slack.

4 Attach the wire to the connecting leads and pacing box.

Check the threshold

1 Set the box to 'demand' mode with a pacing rate faster than the intrinsic heart rate. Set the output at 3 V. This should result in paced rhythm.

2 If it does not, you need to find a better position. Before moving from a position that may have taken a long while to achieve, make sure all connections are secure.

3 Progressively reduce the output until there is failure to capture: the heart rate drops abruptly and pacing spikes are seen but not followed by paced beats (Fig. 53.4). A threshold of <1 V is acceptable. A threshold a little above this is acceptable if it is stable and if the procedure has been difficult or if there is a large infarct or other factors expected to cause a high threshold (Table 53.2).

4 Check the stability of the wire. Set the box at a rate faster than the intrinsic heart rate, with an output of 1 V. Ask the patient to cough forcefully, sniff, and breathe deeply. Watch the monitor for loss of capture.

Placement of flotation pacing wire without screening

1 Hold the electrode above the chest wall in the approximate shape in which it is expected to lie. Note the proximal marker which is level with the hub of the central cannula.

■ **Table 53.2** Causes of failure to capture and/or sense

- Wire malpositioned or displaced
- Ventricular perforation
- Myocardial fibrosis (from previous infarction or cardiomyopathy)
- Drugs (class I anti-arrhythmics)
- Lead contacts not secure

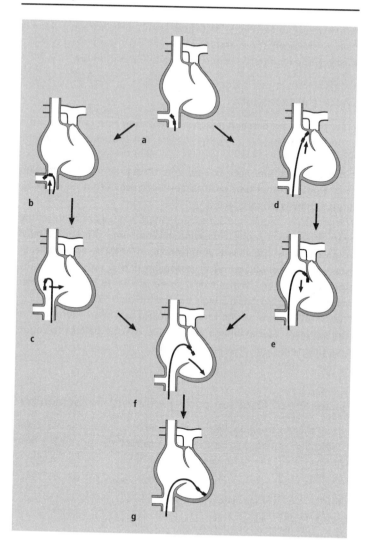

2 Check that the balloon inflates and deflates easily.

3 Insert the pacing wire with the balloon deflated. As soon as it is judged to be beyond the tip of the sheath, inflate the balloon. Insert to the previously noted marker then deflate the balloon.

4 Attach the pacing leads and box.

5 Check threshold as above.

Final points

1 Set the output at more than three times the threshold or 3 V whichever is higher. Set the mode to 'demand'. If in sinus rhythm, set a back-up rate of 50/min. If there is heart block or bradycardia, set at 70–80/min.

2 Removing the insertion sheath reduces the risk of lead displacement, but makes this complication more difficult to correct should it occur.

3 Suture the wire to the skin close to the point of insertion and cover it with a dressing. The rest of the wire should be looped and fixed to the skin with adhesive tape.

4 Obtain a chest X-ray to confirm a satisfactory position of the wire and exclude a pneumothorax.

Aftercare

1 Check the pacing threshold daily. The threshold usually rises to

Fig. 53.2 (*Opposite*) Placement of a ventricular pacing wire from the inferior vena cava (via femoral vein): **a**, catheter is advanced to the hepatic vein; **b**, catheter tip engages proximal hepatic vein and is advanced further; **c**, a loop or bend is formed in the distal catheter, which is then rotated medially; **d**, alternatively, the catheter is advanced to the high-medial right atrium; **e**, with advancement, a bend is formed in the catheter, which is then quickly withdrawn or 'snapped' back to the level of the tricuspid orifice; **f**, after crossing the tricuspid valve, the catheter is advanced with counterclockwise torque to avoid the interventricular septum; **g**, final catheter position in the right ventricular apex. Catheter positions in c and d can be used for atrial pacing. From Ellenbogen KA, ed. *Cardiac Pacing.* Boston: Blackwell Scientific Publications, 1992; 178–9.

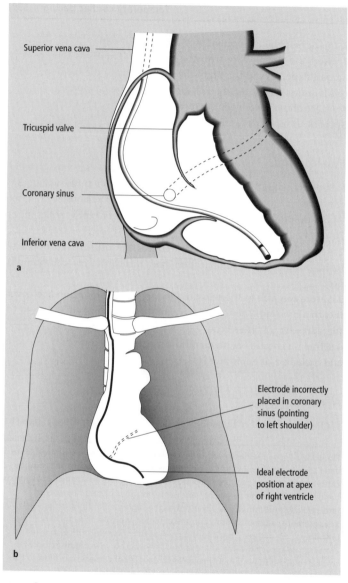

Fig. 53.3 Lead position for temporary ventricular pacing: **a**, anatomy; **b**, screening.

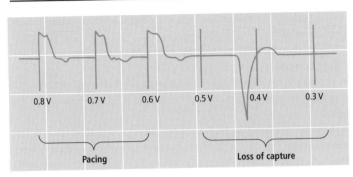

Fig. 53.4 Determination of pacing threshold. The voltage is progressively reduced until there is loss of capture. The vertical lines are pacing artefacts. From Rothman MT. *Hospital Update* 1981; June: 645.

two-to-three times its initial value over the first few days after insertion.

2 If infection related to the wire is suspected see p. 321.

Troubleshooting

Tachyarrhythmias

• Ventricular extrasystoles and non-sustained ventricular tachycardia (VT) are common as the wire crosses the tricuspid valve and do not require treatment.

• If non-sustained VT recurs, check that the position of the wire is still satisfactory and that excess slack has not formed in the area of the tricuspid valve.

Failure to capture and/or sense (Table 53.2)

• The threshold normally increases by a factor of about three after insertion because of endocardial oedema.

- The commonest reason for failure to capture and/or sense is wire displacement.
- Check that the wire tip is pointing downwards at the apex of the right ventricle.
- A position in an epicardial vein looks similar to the correct one, but the wire may be seen more easily and tends to curve round at the apex.
- A wire misplaced in the coronary sinus points towards the left shoulder (see Fig. 53.3) and tends to move as a whole and away from the cardiac apex during systole (because it lies in the atrioventricular groove).
- If a threshold < 1 V cannot be found after trying alternative sites, accept a high threshold in a stable position.

Perforation

1 Suspect with:
   - failure to capture and/or sense;
   - pericardial chest pain;
   - diaphragmatic pacing at low output.
2 Are there signs of cardiac tamponade (p. 148)? If so arrange urgent echocardiography and pericardial drainage.
3 Reposition or replace the wire.

Pericardial rub

This may occur in the absence of perforation. Check the threshold and for signs of tamponade.

Pacing of the diaphragm

This may occur with normal lead position at high output (10 V), but otherwise suggests cardiac perforation (see above).

54 Pericardial aspiration

1 **Cardiac tamponade** (p. 148). Echocardiography must be done first to confirm the presence of a pericardial effusion unless there is cardiac arrest from presumed tamponade.

2 **Pericardial effusion due to suspected bacterial pericarditis** (p. 146).
  - **Aspiration should only be attempted if the effusion is large** (echo separation > 2 cm).
  - **Diagnostic pericardial aspiration is otherwise rarely indicated:** if you are considering this, seek expert advice first from a cardiologist.
  - **Pericardial aspiration may have life-threatening complications** (Table 54.1).

Special equipment

1 **Long needle** (15 cm, 18G) **or long 'cannula-over-needle' IV cannula** (e.g. Wallace).

2 **Guidewire** (80 cm or more, 0.035 inches diameter, with J-end).

3 **Dilator** (5–7 French).

4 **Pigtail catheter** (60-cm long, 5–7 French diameter, multiple sideholes).

5 **Drainage bag and connector.**

■ **Table 54.1** Complications of pericardial aspiration

- Vasovagal reaction
- Penetration of a cardiac chamber (usually right ventricle) – may result in acute tamponade
- Laceration of a coronary artery – may result in acute tamponade
- Arrhythmia
- Pneumothorax
- Perforation of stomach or colon

Technique

Preparation

1 Arrange either X-ray or echocardiographic screening.

2 Lay the patient semirecumbent in the screening room and propped up so the effusion pools anteriorly and inferiorly. Connect an ECG monitor. Ensure you have venous access. Take blood for group and save. Ensure that resuscitation equipment including a defibrillator is to hand. Give sedation with midazolam (2 mg (elderly 1 mg) IV over

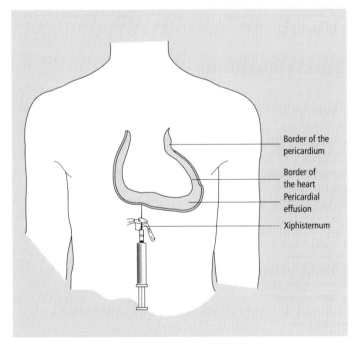

Border of the pericardium

Border of the heart

Pericardial effusion

Xiphisternum

Fig. 54.1 Pericardial aspiration.

30 s, followed after 2 min by increments of 0.5–1 mg if sedation not adequate; usual range 2.5–7.5 mg).

3 Put on gown, mask and gloves. Prepare the skin from midchest to midabdomen and put on drapes.

4 Anaesthetize the skin from a point in the midline (within 5 cm below the xiphisternum) along a track running just below the costal margin towards the head (Fig. 54.1).

5 Make a small skin incision.

Insertion of the catheter

1 Attach the long needle or cannula-over-needle to a 10 ml syringe containing lignocaine and advance it slowly along the anaesthetized track aiming for the suprasternal notch. Angle it at about 30° so that it passes just under the costal margin. Every centimetre or so, aspirate and inject some lignocaine.

2 As soon as fluid is aspirated, remove the syringe and introduce about 20 cm of the guidewire (if you are using a cannula-over-needle, the needle will have to be withdrawn first). See **Troubleshooting** if there is doubt as to whether the fluid is pericardial effusion or blood.

3 Check the position of the guidewire by screening. It should loop freely within the cardiac shadow.

4 Dilate the track.

5 Introduce the pigtail catheter over the guidewire. Keep the guidewire taut and whilst screening, push the catheter through the pericardium and about 20 cm into the pericardial cavity. If a pigtail is not available, fluid can be aspirated through the sheath of a large Seldinger-type central venous cannula.

6 Take specimens for microscopy, culture and cytology. Then aspirate to dryness.

7 Insert a skin suture and loop it over the catheter several times tieing it each time. Attach the connector and drainage bag via a three-way tap. Fix securely with adhesive tape.

Troubleshooting

You cannot enter the effusion

- Consider the apical or left parasternal routes, but check first with echocardiography that there is sufficient fluid and no lung along the proposed needle track.

The pigtail catheter will not pass over the guidewire into the pericardial space

- Check that the guidewire is correctly positioned within the cardiac shadow.
- Check that the guidewire is held taut and not looped.
- Use a larger dilator.

You aspirate heavily blood-stained fluid

1 The possibilities are:
- haemorrhagic effusion (common in malignancy or Dressler's syndrome);
- venous puncture;
- right heart puncture;
- laceration of a coronary artery with haemopericardium.

2 Keep hold of the needle, but remove the syringe and empty into a clean pot. Blood will clot, but even heavily blood-stained effusion will not.

3 Remove 5 ml more fluid and reinject whilst imaging using echocardiography. The cavity containing the needle tip will be marked by microbubbles.

4 If you are still in doubt, compare the haematocrit of the fluid with that of a venous sample (both sent in EDTA tubes), or connect to a pressure monitor: right ventricular penetration is shown by a characteristic waveform (Fig. 52.2, p. 326).

55 DC countershock

Indications

Conversion of ventricular and supraventricular tachyarrhythmias.

Technique

Ventricular fibrillation or pulseless ventricular tachycardia

Give immediate unsynchronized countershock, starting at 200 J (p. 5).

Other tachyarrhythmias

Preparation

1 If this is an elective procedure for atrial flutter or fibrillation, check that the patient is appropriately prepared (Table 55.1).

2 Check that cardioversion is warranted. Fast atrial fibrillation in a patient with mitral valve disease or impaired myocardial function is unlikely to respond and is better treated by digitalization (p. 20). Tachyarrhythmias caused by digoxin toxicity should be treated conservatively (nodal or atrial tachycardia) or initially with lignocaine (ventricular tachycardia).

3 Contact an anaesthetist. A brief general anaesthetic is preferable to sedation with a benzodiazepine.

4 Record a 12-lead ECG.

5 Change the leads from the bedside to the defibrillator monitor. Adjust the leads until the R waves are significantly higher than the T waves and check that the synchronizing marker falls consistently on the QRS complex and not the T wave.

6 Put in a peripheral venous cannula. Check that resuscitation equipment and drugs are to hand.

■ **Table 55.1** Checklist before elective DC cardioversion of atrial flutter or fibrillation

Nil by mouth

- For at least 4 hours before the procedure

Anticoagulation

- Anticoagulation is not necessary for pure atrial flutter or for atrial fibrillation reliably known to be of less than 2 days duration
- If the patient has been in atrial fibrillation for more than 2 days, ensure that warfarin anticoagulation has been given for at least 3 weeks, with INR > 2.0. Check that the current INR is > 2.0

Plasma potassium

- Check that this is > 3.5 mmol/l

Plasma digoxin

- Check that there are no features to suggest toxicity (nausea, xanthopsia, slow AF, frequent ventricular extrasystoles), and that if the dose is high (> 0.25 mg/day) renal function is normal

Thyroid function

- In patients with AF, check that thyroid function is normal: cardioversion of AF due to thyrotoxicosis (which may be otherwise occult) is unlikely to be successful

Suspected brady–tachy syndrome

- Consider inserting a temporary pacing wire because asystole or severe bradycardia may complicate DC cardioversion

AF, Atrial fibrillation; INR, International Normalized Ratio.

Cardioversion

1 One paddle is placed on a pad of jelly over the sternum and the other over the apex.

2 If digoxin toxicity is possible, use a low initial charge and consider giving lignocaine 100 mg before countershock. Initial charges are given in Table 55.2.

■ **Table 55.2** Initial charge for DC countershock

	Initial charge	Mode*
Ventricular fibrillation/pulseless ventricular tachycardia	200 J	Unsynchronized
Ventricular tachycardia	200 J	Synchronized
Atrial fibrillation	50 J	Synchronized
Other supraventricular arrhythmias	25 J	Synchronized
Loaded with digoxin or digoxin toxicity possible	10–20 J	Synchronized

*In synchronized mode, the machine will not discharge until it senses an R wave, to ensure that the shock is delivered during and not after the QRS complex.

3 If this fails, double the power level (unless the procedure is elective and has been followed by prolonged sinus pause or ventricular arrhythmia).

Aftercare
1 Record a 12-lead ECG.
2 Consider prophylactic anti-arrhythmic therapy (Chapter 2).
3 Continue warfarin anticoagulation in patients with atrial fibrillation for at least 3 weeks because atrial mechanical activity may not recover for several days after reversion to sinus rhythm. If there is significant mitral stenosis, anticoagulation should be permanent because the risk of reversion is high.
4 Apply hydrocortisone cream to avoid painful dermatitis.

56 Insertion of a chest drain

Preparation

1 Check the position of the effusion or pneumothorax by examination and on the chest X-ray (ensure you have not misdiagnosed an emphysematous bulla, p. 179).

2 Assemble the underwater seal (Fig. 56.1) and check that the connections fit.

3 Choose the largest tube (usually 28 Ch.) that is likely to fit the intercostal space.

4 Position the patient lying flat or semirecumbent with the hand resting behind the neck.

5 For a pneumothorax, the best approach is usually the third or fourth space in the midaxillary line. This is less alarming for the patient and there is less muscle to be crossed than with the second space in the midclavicular line. The apical approach is dangerous and should not be used. For drainage of an effusion or empyema, the best position can be determined by ultrasound examination, but try to use a midaxillary approach if practical.

6 Prepare and drape the skin.

Insertion of the tube

1 Draw up 20 ml of lignocaine 1%. With the smallest available needle infiltrate the skin with about 2–3 ml then change to a green (21 G) needle. Advance the needle into the thorax until air (or effusion fluid) is aspirated then withdraw slightly and infiltrate about 5 ml around the pleura, leaving a further 2–3 ml in the needle track as you withdraw.

2 Make a 1-cm incision with a scalpel in line with and just above the edge of the lower rib of the intercostal space. With a small Spencer–

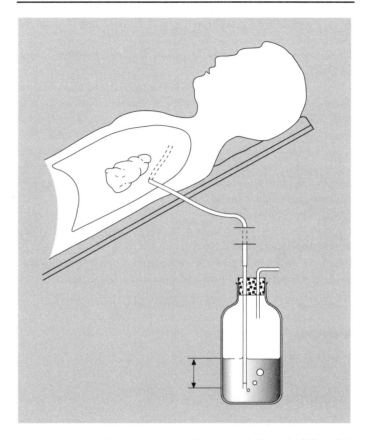

Fig. 56.1 Insertion of a chest drain: underwater seal. The end of the tube is 2–3 cm below the level of the water in the bottle. If intrapleural pressure rises above 2–3 cm water, air will bubble out. If intrapleural pressure becomes negative, water rises up the tube only to fall again when intrapleural pressure falls towards atmospheric. The system operates as a simple one-way valve. When the pneumothorax has resolved, the water level will generally be slightly negative throughout the respiratory cycle and reflect the normal fluctuation in intrapleural pressure, and when the patient coughs air will no longer bubble out. From Brewis RAL. *Lecture Notes on Respiratory Disease*. 3rd edn. Oxford: Blackwell Scientific Publications, 1985; 290.

Wells or similar forceps, enlarge the track down to and through the pleura.

3 Insert a purse string suture of 1/0 silk around the incision taking deep bites.

4 It should now be possible to slide the trochar and tube into the thoracic cavity with virtually no force. If you find that you have to push, withdraw the trochar and enlarge the track. As the trochar enters the pleural space, withdraw it as you advance the tube.

5 For a pneumothorax, direct the tube towards the apex of the thoracic cavity, until about 25 cm of drain are within the chest. The sideholes on the tube must be well within the thoracic cavity or subcutaneous emphysema will result.

6 Attach the underwater seal.

7 Secure the tube with a second 1/0 silk suture wrapped and tied several times around the drain.

8 Coil the ends of the purse-string beneath a pad of gauze placed between the skin and the tube and strap in place with adhesive tape (Fig. 56.2).

Aftercare

● See Fig. 56.2.

Troubleshooting

Pain

Pain around the chest incision may occur. Non-steroidal anti-inflammatory drugs are usually effective, but initially opiates may be needed. If the pain is more distant, you should check the position of the cannula tip. If it is curled against the interior of the thoracic cavity, withdraw it slightly. There should be about 25 cm of intrathoracic tube in an adult of normal size.

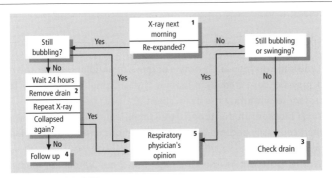

EXPLANATORY NOTES

1 Chest X-ray If the underwater seal is *always* kept below the level of the chest, clamping is unnecessary and potentially dangerous. As far as possible, an X-ray film should be taken in the department, rather than on the ward with a portable machine; an expiration film is unnecessary.

2 Removal of chest drain Bubbling should have stopped for at least 24 hours. Since some patients find tube removal unpleasant, consider premedication . After removing the suture that holds the drain in place, withdraw the tube while the patient holds his or her breath in full inspiration. Use the two remaining sutures to seal the wound.

3 Check chest drain If the lung has not reinflated but there is no bubbling in the underwater bottle, then the tube is blocked or kinked—this can be corrected; or else the tube has become displaced—a replacement must be inserted through a clean incision.

4 Follow up Arrange for a chest clinic appointment in 7–10 days. The patient must be given a discharge letter and told to attend again immediately in the event of noticeable deterioration. Air travel should be avoided until changes seen on radiographs have resolved.

5 Respiratory physician's opinion Should advice from a specialist be required, transfer of continuing care is advisable. Important considerations in management are:
• assessing why re-expansion has not been achieved (for example, air leaking around the drain site, tube displaced or blocked, large persistent leak);
• the use of suction to re-expand the lung (this can be lengthy, requires appropriate equipment and pressure settings, influences how and where confirmatory radiographs are taken, and involves care from experienced nursing staff);
• whether early thoracic surgery would be appropriate (for example, failure of conservative measures, need to prevent recurrence);
• consideration of chemical pleurodesis in certain cases;
• management of surgical emphysema.

Fig. 56.2 Management of intercostal drain. From Miller AC, Harvey JE. *BMJ* 1993; 307: 114–6.

Fluid level does not swing with breathing

- **Tube kinked:** this usually occurs because of angulation over the ribs and may be corrected by releasing the dressing. Occasionally it is necessary to withdraw the drain slightly.
- **Tube blocked:** if the tube is too small, which is the commonest fault, it can easily become blocked by secretions. It should be replaced by a larger one.
- **Wrong position:** if the drainage holes are wholly or partially extrapleural, which can be diagnosed from the chest film, the tube needs to be removed and another replaced.

Surgical emphysema

A little localized subcutaneous air is usual, but increasing surgical emphysema indicates malposition of the tube with a drainage hole in a subcutaneous position. A new tube must be inserted.

Pneumothorax does not resolve

If the tube is well positioned, of adaquate size (the largest that can be comfortably inserted) and not blocked, this indicates a persisting bronchopleural fistula. Seek expert advice from a chest physician or thoracic surgeon. Some will resolve with low-pressure suction.

57 Lumbar puncture

Indications

1 Suspected meningitis (p. 204).
2 Suspected subarachnoid haemorrhage (p. 200).
3 Suspected Guillain–Barré syndrome (p. 214).
NB: If you suspect bacterial meningitis, take blood cultures and start antibiotic therapy immediately (p. 205), before performing lumbar puncture (LP).

Contraindications

1 Reduced level of consciousness.
2 Focal neurological signs (long tract or posterior fossa).
3 Papilloedema.
4 Anticoagulation.
LP may be performed in patients with contraindications, but not before obtaining expert advice from a neurologist or neurosurgeon.

Special equipment

1 Spinal needle. The disposable ones are usually sharper. Choose a 20 or 22 G needle.
2 Manometer and three-way tap.
3 Three plain sterile bottles (numbered) and a fluoride bottle for glucose (to be sent with a blood glucose sample, taken before LP).

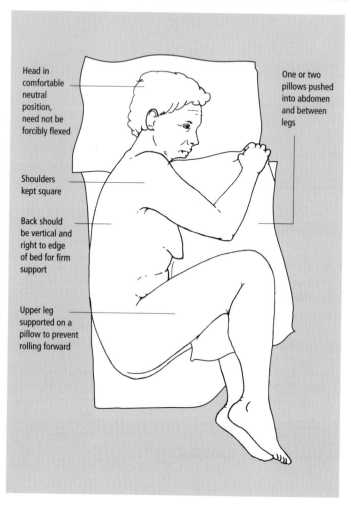

Head in comfortable neutral position, need not be forcibly flexed

One or two pillows pushed into abdomen and between legs

Shoulders kept square

Back should be vertical and right to edge of bed for firm support

Upper leg supported on a pillow to prevent rolling forward

Fig. 57.1 Positioning the patient for LP. From Patten J. *Neurological Differential Diagnosis.* London: Harold Starke, 1977; 262.

Technique

Positioning the patient (Fig. 57.1)

1 Move the patient to the edge of the bed, on their left side if you are right-handed.

2 The thoracolumbar spine should be maximally flexed. It does not matter if the neck is not flexed. Place a pillow between the knees to prevent torsion of the spine.

Choose the interspace to be used

1 Define the plane of the iliac crests, which runs through L3−4. The spinal cord in the adult ends at the level of L1−2.

2 Choose either the L3−4 or L4−5 spaces. Mark the space using your thumbnail.

Lumbar puncture

1 Put on gloves and prepare the skin. It helps to place a drape on top of the patient so that you can recheck the position of the iliac crest if necessary.

2 Draw up lignocaine, assemble the manometer and undo the tops of the bottles. Check that the stylet of the needle moves freely. Place everything within easy reach.

3 Stretch the skin over the chosen space with the finger and thumb of your left hand, placed on the spinous processes of the adjacent vertebrae (Fig. 57.2). Put 0.5 ml of lignocaine in the skin and sub-cutaneous tissues with an orange needle.

4 Place the spinal needle on the mark, bevel uppermost, and advance it towards the umbilicus, taking care to keep it parallel to the ground.

5 The interspinous ligament gives some resistance, and you should notice increased resistance as you go through the tough ligamentum flavum. There is usually an obvious 'give' when the needle is through

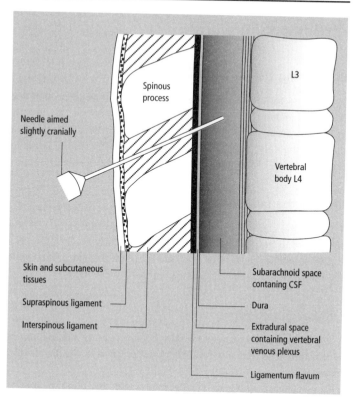

Fig. 57.2 The anatomy of LP.

this. The dura is now only 1–2 mm away. Advance in small steps, withdrawing the stylet after each step.

6 Cerebrospinal fluid (CSF) should flow freely once you enter the dura. If the flow is poor, rotate the needle in case a nerve root is lying against it.

Measuring the opening pressure and collecting cerebrospinal fluid

1 Connect the manometer and measure the height of the CSF column

(the 'opening pressure'). The patient should uncurl slightly and try to relax at this stage.

2 Cap the top of the manometer with your finger, disconnect it from the needle and put the CSF in the glucose tube.

3 Collect three samples (about 2 ml each) in the plain sterile bottles.

4 Remove the needle and place a small dressing over the puncture site.

Interpreting cerebrospinal fluid results

• Normal values are given in Table 57.1, and CSF formulae in meningitis in Table 57.2.

Problems

You hit bone

1 Withdraw the needle. Recheck the patient's position and the bony landmarks. Try again, taking particular care to keep the needle parallel to the ground.

2 If this fails, modify the angle of the needle in the sagittal plane.

3 If you are still unsuccessful, try another space.

■ **Table 57.1** Cerebrospinal fluid: normal values and correction for traumatic tap

Opening pressure	7–18 cm CSF
Cell count	0–5 mm^3, all lymphocytes
Protein concentration	0.15–0.45 g/l (15–45 mg/dl)
Glucose concentration	2.8–4.2 mmol/l
CSF:blood glucose ratio	>50%

Traumatic tap – correction of cell count and protein concentration: for every 1000 RBC/mm^3 subtract 1 WBC/mm^3 and 0.015 g/l (1.5 mg/dl) protein.

References:

Normal reference values. *N Engl J Med* 1986; 314: 39–49.

Gottlieb AJ, Zamkoff KW, Jastremski MS, Scalzo A, Imboden KJ. *The Whole Internist Catalog.* Philadelphia: WB Saunders, 1980: 127–8.

■ **Table 57.2** Cerebrospinal fluid formulae in meningitis

	Pyogenic	Viral	Tuberculous	Cryptococcal
Cell count/mm^3	> 1000	< 500	< 500	< 150
Predominant cell type	Polymorphs	Lymphocytes	Lymphocytes	Lymphocytes
Protein concentration (g/l)	> 1.5	0.5 − 1	1 − 5	0.5 − 1
CSF : blood glucose	< 50%	> 50%	< 50%	< 50%

• The values given are typical, but many exceptions occur.
• Antibiotic therapy substantially changes the CSF formula in pyogenic bacterial meningitis, leading to a fall in cell count, increased proportion of lymphocytes and fall in protein level. However, the low CSF glucose level usually persists.

Heavily blood-stained fluid

1 The possibilities are subarachnoid haemorrhage, traumatic tap or puncture of the venous plexus. If the fluid appears to be venous blood (slow ooze) try again in another space, after flushing the needle.
2 Subarachnoid haemorrhage results in uniformly blood-stained CSF (as shown by the red-cell count in successive samples). Xanthochromia of the supernatant is always found from 12 hours to 2 weeks after the bleed; centrifuge the CSF and examine the supernatant by spectrophotometry.

Deteriorating conscious level after lumbar puncture

1 Give mannitol 20% 100−200 ml (0.5 g/kg) IV over 10 min. Check plasma osmolality: further mannitol may be given until plasma osmolality is 320 mosmol/kg.
2 Arrange transfer to the intensive-therapy unit in case intubation

and ventilation are needed. If intubated, hyperventilate to a $Pa\text{CO}_2$ of 4.0 kPa (30 mmHg).

3 Seek expert advice on further management from a neurologist or neurosurgeon.

58 Peritoneal dialysis

Indications

- **Acute renal failure**, when other methods of renal replacement therapy are not possible or are contraindicated.
- **Elimination of some poisons** (e.g. lithium), when haemodialysis is not possible.
- **Core rewarming in hypothermia** (p. 279).

Contraindications

- **Recent abdominal surgery**
- **Hypercatabolic states**

Technique

Preparation

1 Prepare a 1-l bag of dialysis fluid warmed to 37°C.
2 Lay the patient flat.
3 Confirm that the bladder is empty by ultrasound, or, if this is not available, by catheterization.
4 Shave the lower abdomen.
5 Put on gown, gloves and mask and prepare and drape the skin.

Inserting the catheter

1 The usual site for insertion is 1 inch below the umbilicus in the midline. If there is an operation scar here, use a more lateral site (avoid the area of the inferior epigastric artery, whose surface marking is a line joining the femoral artery with the umbilicus).

2 Infiltrate with 10−15 ml of lignocaine 1% down to and around the peritoneum.

3 Aspirate for gas (indicating perforation of bowel) and if found, choose another site.

4 Insert an IV cannula into the peritoneal cavity and run in the prepared dialysis fluid using a standard IV-giving set. Withdraw the cannula. (This step is optional but makes inserting the peritoneal dialysis (PD) catheter easier.)

5 Incise the skin vertically with a narrow scalpel blade (e.g. No. 11) and insert the PD catheter through the abdominal wall with a twisting action.

6 As soon as the tip is through the peritoneum (signalled by loss of resistance), rotate the catheter so that the black spot (which marks the direction of the curve) is facing inferolaterally. Withdraw the obturator 2 cm. Advance the catheter, aiming downwards and laterally towards the pelvis, until two-thirds has been inserted. Then withdraw the obturator completely as you advance the catheter until only 2 cm is protruding.

7 Attach the right-angled end of the connecting set to the catheter, which should be held with a deep purse-string suture (3/0 silk).

8 Place gauze swabs around the catheter. Use a split gallipot to support it and the connecting piece if kinking could occur.

Peritoneal dialysis for acute renal failure

Choice of fluid

- PD fluid is available in 1- or 2-l bags. The osmolality of the fluid (which influences the shift of water from plasma to PD fluid) varies according to the dextrose concentration.
- Start with 1-l bags of 1.36% dextrose unless the patient is fluid-overloaded in which case use dextrose of a higher concentration.

Exchanges

1 Weigh the bags before and after use to calculate their fluid capacity (allow 1 ml/g) as they may not contain exactly 1 l.

2 Warm the fluid to 37°C. Add heparin (500 U/l) to reduce fibrin deposition on the catheter.

3 The exchange time consists of inflow time, dwell time and outflow time. Start with hourly exchanges, roughly 20 min each for inflow, dwell and outflow. If inflow and outflow take longer, omit the dwell time.

4 The exchange time can be increased after the first day if the patient's biochemistry and fluid status is satisfactory.

5 If plasma potassium falls below 3.5 mmol/l, potassium should be added to the PD fluid to give a concentration of 4 mmol/l.

Monitoring (Table 58.1)

Check plasma potassium 4 hours after starting dialysis and then at least twice daily.

■ **Table 58.1** Monitoring the patient during peritoneal dialysis

Hourly

- Inflow volume estimated by weight
- Volume of effluent
- Volume of other fluid in or out

4-hourly

- Temperature
- Pulse and BP

8–12 hourly

- Stick test for glucose. Some patients develop hyperglycaemia particularly when hyperosmolar PD fluid is used
- Plasma biochemistry

Daily
- Weight after drainage of PD fluid

Peritoneal dialysis for core rewarming in hypothermia

Choice of fluid

- Use 1- or 2-l bags, potassium free.
- Warm the dialysate by running it through a blood-warming coil immersed in water heated to 54°C: this will give a dialysate temperature around 44°C when it enters the peritoneal cavity.

Exchanges

Run in rapidly and drain out immediately. Core temperature is usually restored to normal after six to eight exchanges.

Monitoring

Check plasma potassium hourly and if < 3.5 mmol/l, add potassium to the dialysate (4 mmol/l).

Troubleshooting

Fluid accumulation/poor drainage

- Accumulation of 500–1000 ml is usual.
- Check that the catheter is not kinked as it leaves the abdomen. Syringe the catheter with saline.
- If fluid accumulation is progressive (often due to plugging of the end of the catheter by omentum), the catheter will have to be resited. The position of the catheter can be checked by ultrasound. Resiting is best done with a second catheter, leaving the first in place to prevent leakage of fluid down the track.

■ **Table 58.2** 'Blind' antibotic therapy for peritonitis complicating peritoneal dialysis

Vancomycin plus gentamicin or **ceftazidime**

Vancomycin

- Loading dose: 500 mg intraperitoneally (IP)
- Maintenance dose: 25 mg/l IP

Gentamicin

- Loading dose: 1.7 mg/kg IP
- Maintenance dose: 4 mg/l IP
- Check a random blood level after 4 days and reduce the dose if this is 4 mg/l or more

Ceftazidime

- 500 mg/l IP

Peritonitis

- Shown by abdominal pain, fever and cloudy effluent.
- Aspirate 30 ml of effluent through the wall or port of the bag (sterilize the site with an alcohol swab).
- Divide 10 ml between aerobic and anaerobic blood culture bottles. Send 20 ml for cell count and centrifugation with Gram staining and culture of the sediment.
- Initial antibiotic therapy is given in Table 58.2.
- Antibiotic treatment should be continued for at least 5 days after clearing of the effluent (usually for a total of 7–10 days).

59 Insertion of a Sengstaken–Blakemore tube

Indication

Failure to control variceal bleeding despite infusion of vasopressin and nitrate (p. 227).

- **Insertion of a Sengstaken–Blakemore tube is rarely necessary and should only be performed for life-threatening haemorrhage.** If you have not had experience of putting in these tubes it is better to manage the patient conservatively because of the risks of inhalation, mucosal ulceration and incorrect positioning.
- **Balloon tamponade is not a definitive procedure.** Plan ahead for variceal injection or oesophageal transection.

Special equipment

1 Sengstaken–Blakemore tube (Fig. 59.1). If this has only three lumens, tape a standard medium-bore nasogastric tube with the perforations just above the oesophageal balloon to allow aspiration of the oesophagus. If there is time, store the tube in the freezer section of a refrigerator to reduce its flexibility to ease insertion.

2 Mercury sphygmomanometer (for inflation of the oesophageal balloon).

3 Contrast medium (e.g. Gastrografin) 10 ml and 300 ml water or 5% dextrose (for inflation of the gastric balloon). Normal saline should not be used as routine because of the potential dangers of sodium ingestion in the presence of hepatic decompensation should the balloon burst.

4 Bladder syringe for aspirating the oesophageal drainage tube.

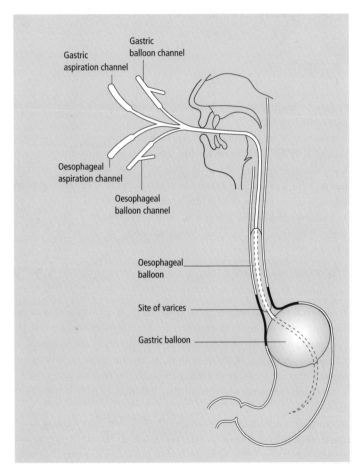

Gastric
aspiration channel

Gastric
balloon channel

Oesophageal
aspiration channel

Oesophageal
balloon channel

Oesophageal
balloon

Site of varices

Gastric balloon

Fig. 59.1 Four-lumen Sengstaken–Blakemore tube in place to compress bleeding varices. From Thompson R. *Lecture Notes on the Liver*. Oxford: Blackwell Scientific Publications, 1985; 37.

Technique

Preparation

1 The lumens of the tube are not always labelled: if they are not, label them now with tape.

2 The patient should be intubated before insertion of the tube (to prevent misplacement of the tube in the trachea or inhalation of blood) if:

- the conscious level is severely depressed; or
- the gag reflex is reduced or absent.

3 Sedation with midazolam (2 mg (elderly 1 mg) IV over 30 s, followed after 2 min by increments of 0.5–1 mg if sedation not adequate; usual range 2.5–7.5 mg) should be used only if the patient is particularly agitated and an anaesthetist is available in case intubation becomes necessary. Some patients may become more agitated after benzodiazepines. To avoid the risk of traumatic insertion, it is safest to intubate and ventilate these patients before insertion is attempted.

Insertion of the tube

1 Anaesthetize the throat with lignocaine spray.

2 Lubricate the end of the tube with KY jelly and pass it through the gap between your index and middle fingers as they are placed in the back of the oropharynx. This reduces the chance of the tube curling. Ask the patient to breathe quietly through the mouth throughout the procedure. You are unlikely to need a chock for the teeth.

3 If at any stage of the procedure the patient becomes dyspnoeic withdraw the tube immediately and start again after endotracheal intubation.

4 Assistants should aspirate blood from the mouth and from all lumens while you insert the tube.

5 Steadily advance the tube until it is inserted to the hilt.

6 Inflate the gastric balloon with the contrast mixture. Insert a bung or

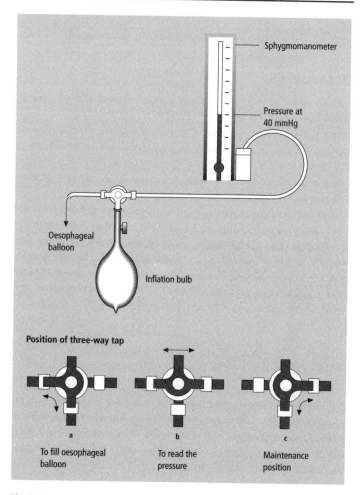

Fig. 59.2 Method of filling the oesophageal balloon and measuring its pressure.

clamp the tube. If there is resistance to inflation, deflate the balloon and check the position of the tube with X-ray screening.

7 Pull the tube back gently until resistance is felt.

8 Firm traction on the gastric balloon is usually sufficient to stop the bleeding as this occurs at the filling point of the varices in the lower few centimetres of the oesophagus. If not, inflate the oesophageal balloon:

- connect the lumen of the oesophageal balloon to a sphygmomanometer via a three-way tap (Fig. 59.2);
- inflate to 40 mmHg and clamp the tube;
- the oesophageal balloon tends to deflate easily so the pressure must be checked every 2 hours or so.

9 Place a sponge pad (as used to support endotracheal tubes in ventilated patients) over the side of the patient's mouth to prevent the tube rubbing.

10 Strap the tube to the cheek. Fixation with weights over the end of the bed is less effective.

11 Mark the tube in relation to the teeth so that movement can be detected more easily.

Aftercare

1 It is not necessary to deflate the oesophageal balloon every hour as sometimes recommended.

2 Continue infusions of vasopressin and nitrate.

3 Obtain a chest X-ray to check the position. The traction applied means that the gastric balloon is usually seen in the thorax.

4 If facilities for variceal injection are available, the tube should be removed in the endoscopy suite immediately prior to injection, which can be done as soon as the patient is haemodynamically stable (usually within 12 hours).

5 If facilities for variceal injection are not available discuss the case with the regional liver unit and arrange transfer if appropriate. Alternatively, start planning for oesophageal transection within 24 hours if bleeding recurs when the balloon is deflated.

6 Do not leave the tube in for longer than 24 hours because of the risk of mucosal ulceration.

7 Changing the side of the attachment to the cheek every 2 hours reduces the risk of skin ulceration, but should be done carefully because of the risk of displacement.

Mistakes to avoid

1 Poor anchoring, or displacement when moving the patient.

2 Failure to plan ahead. Seek expert advice from a gastroenterologist regarding a definitive procedure (variceal injection, oesophageal transection, shunt or embolization).

3 Using air instead of contrast, which allows easy deflation of the balloon with consequent displacement of the tube.

4 Aspiration of blood or endotracheal placement of the tube. You should have a low threshold for intubation and ventilation.

Section 4
Useful Information

60 Drugs and drug infusions

Administration of the following drugs is dealt with in this chapter:
1 **adrenaline and noradrenaline;**
2 **dobutamine;**
3 **dopamine;**
4 **heparin;**
5 **warfarin.**
Drug infusions detailed elsewhere are given in Table 60.1.

■ **Table 60.1** Guide to drug infusions

Drug	Indication	Page reference
Acetylcysteine	Paracetamol poisoning	102
Aminophylline	Bronchospasm	164
Amiodarone	Treatment of VF/VT	20
Chlormethiazole	Alcohol withdrawal	71
Doxapram	Respiratory failure	170
Insulin	Diabetes	264
Isoprenaline	Bradycardia	22
Labetalol	Severe hypertension	134
Lignocaine	Treatment of VF/VT	14
Naloxone	Opiate antagonism	54
Nitroprusside	Severe hypertension	134
Salbutamol	Bronchospasm	164
Trimetaphan	Aortic dissection	131

VF, Ventricular fibrillation; VT, ventricular tachycardia.

Adrenaline and noradrenaline

■ **Table 60.2** Relative inotropic, vasopressor and vasodilator effects of adrenergic agonists

Drug	Inotropic (beta-1)	Vasopressor (alpha-1)	Vasodilator (beta-2)
Adrenaline	3+	1–2+*	3+
Noradrenaline	3+	3+	1+
Dobutamine	3+	0–1+*	1+
Dopamine	2–3+*	0–3+*	2+

Potency expressed using a semiquantitative scale, 0 = no effect, 3+ = marked effect.

* Dose-dependent effect.

■ **Table 60.3** Guide to dosage of adrenergic agonists and enoximone

Drug	Dosage (µg/kg/min)	Comment
Adrenaline	0.05	Beta-1 inotropic and beta-2 vasodilator effects
	0.05–5	Alpha-1 vasoconstriction seen (vasopressor)
Noradrenaline	0.05–5	
Dobutamine	5–40	
Dopamine	2.5	Splanchnic (renal) vasodilatation
	5–10	Beta-1 mediated inotropic effect
	10–40	Alpha-1 mediated vasoconstriction (vasopressor)
Enoximone	2.5–10	Give loading dose of 0.5–0.75 mg/ kg over 5 min first

Adrenaline, noradrenaline and dopamine must be given via a central vein.

■ Table 60.4 Adrenaline and noradrenaline infusions: 2 mg in 50 ml (40 µg/ml)

Infusion volumes (ml/hour)

Dose (µg/kg/min)	Weight (kg) 30	35	40	45	50	55	60	65	70	75	80	85	90	95	100	105	110	115	120
0.01	0.45	0.53	0.6	0.68	0.75	0.83	0.9	0.98	1.05	1.13	1.2	1.28	1.35	1.43	1.5	1.58	1.65	1.73	1.8
0.02	0.9	1.05	1.2	1.35	1.5	1.65	1.8	1.95	2.1	2.25	2.4	2.55	2.7	2.85	3	3.15	3.3	3.45	3.6
0.03	1.35	1.57	1.8	2.02	2.25	2.48	2.7	2.92	3.15	3.38	3.6	3.82	4.05	4.28	4.5	4.72	4.95	5.17	5.4
0.04	1.8	2.1	2.4	2.7	3	3.3	3.6	3.9	4.2	4.5	4.8	5.1	5.4	5.7	6	6.3	6.6	6.9	7.2
0.05	2.25	2.63	3	3.38	3.75	4.13	4.5	4.88	5.25	5.63	6	6.38	6.75	7.13	7.5	7.88	8.25	8.63	9
0.06	2.7	3.15	3.6	4.05	4.5	4.95	5.4	5.85	6.3	6.75	7.2	7.65	8.1	8.55	9	9.45	9.9	10.4	10.8
0.07	3.15	3.68	4.2	4.73	5.25	5.78	6.3	6.83	7.35	7.88	8.4	8.93	9.45	9.98	10.5	11	11.6	12.1	12.6
0.08	3.6	4.2	4.8	5.4	6	6.6	7.2	7.8	8.4	9	9.6	10.2	10.8	11.4	12	12.6	13.2	13.8	14.4
0.09	4.05	4.72	5.4	6.08	6.75	7.42	8.1	8.78	9.45	10.1	10.8	11.5	12.2	12.8	13.5	14.2	14.9	15.5	16.2
0.1	4.5	5.25	6	6.75	7.5	8.25	9	9.75	10.5	11.3	12	12.8	13.5	14.3	15	15.8	16.5	17.3	18
0.2	9	10.5	12	13.5	15	16.5	18	19.5	21	22.5	24	25.5	27	28.5	30	31.5	33	34.5	36

Continued on p. 376

■ **Table 60.4** (Continued)

Infusion volumes (ml/hour)

Dose (µg/kg/min)	Weight (kg) 30	35	40	45	50	55	60	65	70	75	80	85	90	95	100	105	110	115	120
0.3	13.5	15.8	18	20.3	22.5	24.8	27	29.3	31.5	33.8	36	38.3	40.5	42.8	45	47.3	49.5	51.8	54
0.4	18	21	24	27	30	33	36	39	42	45	48	51	54	57	60	63	66	69	72
0.5	22.5	26.3	30	33.8	37.5	41.3	45	48.8	52.5	56.3	60	63.8	67.5	71.3	75	78.8	82.5	86.3	90
0.6	27	31.5	36	40.5	45	49.5	54	58.5	63	67.5	72	76.5	81	85.5	90	94.5	99	104	108
0.7	31.5	36.8	42	47.3	52.5	57.8	63	68.3	73.5	78.8	84	89.3	94.5	99.8	105	110	116	121	126
0.8	36	42	48	54	60	66	72	78	84	90	96	102	108	114	120	126	132	138	144
0.9	40.5	47.3	54	60.8	67.5	74.3	81	87.8	94.5	101	108	115	122	128	135	142	149	155	162
1	45	52.5	60	67.5	75	82.5	90	97.5	105	113	120	128	135	143	150	158	165	173	180

■ **Table 60.5** Adrenaline and noradrenaline infusions: 4 mg in 50 ml (80 µg/ml)

Infusion volumes (ml/hour)

Dose (µg/kg/min)	Weight (kg) 30	35	40	45	50	55	60	65	70	75	80	85	90	95	100	105	110	115	120
0.01	0.23	0.26	0.3	0.34	0.38	0.41	0.45	0.49	0.53	0.56	0.6	0.64	0.68	0.71	0.75	0.79	0.83	0.86	0.9
0.02	0.45	0.53	0.6	0.68	0.75	0.83	0.9	0.98	1.05	1.13	1.2	1.28	1.35	1.43	1.5	1.58	1.65	1.73	1.8
0.03	0.68	0.79	0.9	1.01	1.13	1.24	1.35	1.46	1.57	1.69	1.8	1.91	2.02	2.14	2.25	2.36	2.48	2.59	2.7
0.04	0.9	1.05	1.2	1.35	1.5	1.65	1.8	1.95	2.1	2.25	2.4	2.55	2.7	2.85	3	3.15	3.3	3.45	3.6
0.05	1.13	1.31	1.5	1.69	1.88	2.06	2.25	2.44	2.63	2.81	3	3.19	3.38	3.56	3.75	3.94	4.13	4.31	4.5
0.06	1.37	1.57	1.8	2.02	2.25	2.48	2.7	2.92	3.15	3.38	3.6	3.82	4.05	4.28	4.5	4.72	4.95	5.17	5.4
0.07	1.58	1.84	2.1	2.36	2.63	2.89	3.15	3.41	3.68	3.94	4.2	4.46	4.73	4.99	5.25	5.51	5.78	6.04	6.3
0.08	1.8	2.1	2.4	2.7	3	3.3	3.6	3.9	4.2	4.5	4.8	5.1	5.4	5.7	6	6.3	6.6	6.9	7.2
0.09	2.02	2.36	2.7	3.04	3.38	3.71	4.05	4.39	4.72	5.06	5.4	5.74	6.08	6.41	6.75	7.09	7.42	7.76	8.1
0.1	2.25	2.63	3	3.38	3.75	4.13	4.5	4.88	5.25	5.63	6	6.38	6.75	7.13	7.5	7.88	8.25	8.63	9
0.2	4.5	5.25	6	6.75	7.5	8.25	9	9.75	10.5	11.3	12	12.8	13.5	14.3	15	15.8	16.5	17.3	18

Continued on p. 378

■ Table 60.5 (Continued)

Infusion volumes (ml/hour)

Dose (µg/kg/min)	Weight (kg) 30	35	40	45	50	55	60	65	70	75	80	85	90	95	100	105	110	115	120
0.3	6.75	7.88	9	10.1	11.3	12.4	13.5	14.6	15.8	16.9	18	19.1	20.3	21.4	22.5	23.6	24.8	25.9	27
0.4	9	10.5	12	13.5	15	16.5	18	19.5	21	22.5	24	25.5	27	28.5	30	31.5	33	34.5	36
0.5	11.3	13.1	15	16.9	18.8	20.6	22.5	24.4	26.3	28.1	30	31.9	33.8	35.6	37.5	39.4	41.3	43.1	45
0.6	13.5	15.8	18	20.3	22.5	24.8	27	29.3	31.5	33.8	36	38.3	40.5	42.8	45	47.3	49.5	51.8	54
0.7	15.8	18.4	21	23.6	26.3	28.9	31.5	34.1	36.8	39.4	42	44.6	47.3	49.9	52.5	55.1	57.8	60.4	63
0.8	18	21	24	27	30	33	36	39	42	45	48	51	54	57	60	63	66	69	72
0.9	20.3	23.6	27	30.4	33.8	37.1	40.5	43.9	47.3	50.6	54	57.4	60.8	64.1	67.5	70.9	74.3	77.6	81
1	22.5	26.3	30	33.8	37.5	41.3	45	48.8	52.5	56.3	60	63.8	67.5	71.3	75	78.8	82.5	86.3	90
2	45	52.5	60	67.5	75	82.5	90	97.5	105	113	120	128	135	143	150	158	165	173	180
3	67.5	78.8	90	101	113	124	135	146	158	169	180	191	203	214	225	236	248	259	270
4	90	105	120	135	150	165	180	195	210	225	240	255	270	285	300	315	330	345	360

■ Table 60.6 Adrenaline and noradrenaline infusions: 8 mg in 50 ml (160 µg/ml)

Infusion volumes (ml/hour)

Dose (µg/kg/min)	Weight (kg) 30	35	40	45	50	55	60	65	70	75	80	85	90	95	100	105	110	115	120
0.1	1.13	1.31	1.5	1.69	1.88	2.06	2.25	2.44	2.63	2.81	3	3.19	3.38	3.56	3.75	3.94	4.13	4.31	4.5
0.2	2.25	2.63	3	3.38	3.75	4.13	4.5	4.88	5.25	5.63	6	6.38	6.75	7.13	7.5	7.88	8.25	8.63	9
0.3	3.38	3.94	4.5	5.06	5.63	6.19	6.75	7.31	7.88	8.44	9	9.56	10.1	10.7	11.3	11.8	12.4	12.9	13.5
0.4	4.5	5.25	6	6.75	7.5	8.25	9	9.75	10.5	11.3	12	12.8	13.5	14.3	15	15.8	16.5	17.3	18
0.5	5.63	6.56	7.5	8.44	9.38	10.3	11.3	12.2	13.1	14.1	15	15.9	16.9	17.8	18.8	19.7	20.6	21.6	22.5
0.6	6.75	7.88	9	10.1	11.3	12.4	13.5	14.6	15.8	16.9	18	19.1	20.3	21.4	22.5	23.6	24.8	25.9	27
0.7	7.88	9.19	10.5	11.8	13.1	14.4	15.8	17.1	18.4	19.7	21	22.3	23.6	24.9	26.3	27.6	28.9	30.2	31.5
0.8	9	10.5	12	13.5	15	16.5	18	19.5	21	22.5	24	25.5	27	28.5	30	31.5	33	34.5	36
0.9	10.1	11.8	13.5	15.2	16.9	18.6	20.3	21.9	23.6	25.3	27	28.7	30.4	32.1	33.8	35.4	37.1	38.8	40.5
1	11.3	13.1	15	16.9	18.8	20.6	22.5	24.4	26.3	28.1	30	31.9	33.8	35.6	37.5	39.4	41.3	43.1	45
2	22.5	26.3	30	33.8	37.5	41.3	45	48.8	52.5	56.3	60	63.8	67.5	71.3	75	78.8	82.5	86.3	90

Continued on p. 380

■ **Table 60.6** *(Continued)*

Infusion volumes (ml/hour)

Dose (µg/kg/min)	Weight (kg) 30	35	40	45	50	55	60	65	70	75	80	85	90	95	100	105	110	115	120
3	33.8	39.4	45	50.6	56.3	61.9	67.5	73.1	78.8	84.4	90	95.6	101	107	113	118	124	129	135
4	45	52.5	60	67.5	75	82.5	90	97.5	105	113	120	128	135	143	150	158	165	173	180
5	56.3	65.6	75	84.4	93.8	103	113	122	131	141	150	159	169	178	188	197	206	216	225
6	67.5	78.8	90	101	113	124	135	146	158	169	180	191	203	214	225	236	248	259	270
7	78.8	91.9	105	118	131	144	158	171	184	197	210	223	236	249	263	276	289	302	315
8	90	105	120	135	150	165	180	195	210	225	240	255	270	285	300	315	330	345	360
9	101	118	135	152	169	186	203	219	236	253	270	287	304	321	338	354	371	388	405
10	113	131	150	169	188	206	225	244	263	281	300	319	338	356	375	394	413	431	405

Dobutamine

■ Table 60.7 Dobutamine infusion: 250 mg in 50 ml (5 mg/ml)

Infusion volumes (ml/hour)

Dose (μg/kg/min)	Weight (kg) 30	35	40	45	50	55	60	65	70	75	80	85	90	95	100	105	110	115	120
1	0.36	0.42	0.48	0.54	0.6	0.66	0.72	0.78	0.84	0.9	0.96	1.02	1.08	1.14	1.2	1.26	1.32	1.38	1.44
2	0.72	0.84	0.96	1.08	1.2	1.32	1.44	1.56	1.68	1.8	1.92	2.04	2.16	2.28	2.4	2.52	2.64	2.76	2.88
3	1.08	1.26	1.44	1.62	1.8	1.98	2.16	2.34	2.52	2.7	2.88	3.06	3.24	3.42	3.6	3.78	3.96	4.14	4.32
4	1.44	1.68	1.92	2.16	2.4	2.64	2.88	3.12	3.36	3.6	3.84	4.08	4.32	4.56	4.8	5.04	5.28	5.52	5.76
5	1.8	2.1	2.4	2.7	3	3.3	3.6	3.9	4.2	4.5	4.8	5.1	5.4	5.7	6	6.3	6.6	6.9	7.2
6	2.16	2.52	2.88	3.24	3.6	3.96	4.32	4.68	5.04	5.4	5.76	6.12	6.48	6.84	7.2	7.56	7.92	8.28	8.64
7	2.52	2.94	3.36	3.78	4.2	4.62	5.04	5.46	5.88	6.3	6.72	7.14	7.56	7.98	8.4	8.82	9.24	9.66	10.1
8	2.88	3.36	3.84	4.32	4.8	5.28	5.76	6.24	6.72	7.2	7.68	8.16	8.64	9.12	9.6	10.1	10.6	11	11.5
9	3.24	3.78	4.32	4.86	5.4	5.94	6.48	7.02	7.56	8.1	8.64	9.18	9.72	10.3	10.8	11.3	11.9	12.4	13

Continued on p. 382

■ Table 60.7 (Continued)

Infusion volumes (ml/hour)

Dose (µg/kg/min)	Weight (kg) 30	35	40	45	50	55	60	65	70	75	80	85	90	95	100	105	110	115	120
10	3.6	4.2	4.8	5.4	6	6.6	7.2	7.8	8.4	9	9.6	10.2	10.8	11.4	12	12.6	13.2	13.8	14.4
20	7.2	8.4	9.6	10.8	12	13.2	14.4	15.6	16.8	18	19.2	20.4	21.6	22.8	24	25.2	26.4	27.6	28.8
30	10.8	12.6	14.4	16.2	18	19.8	21.6	23.4	25.2	27	28.8	30.6	32.4	34.2	36	37.8	39.6	41.4	43.2
40	14.4	16.8	19.2	21.6	24	26.4	28.8	31.2	33.6	36	38.4	40.8	43.2	45.6	48	50.4	52.8	55.2	57.6
50	18	21	24	27	30	33	36	39	42	45	48	51	54	57	60	63	66	69	72
60	21.6	25.2	28.8	32.4	36	39.6	43.2	46.8	50.4	54	57.6	61.2	64.8	68.4	72	75.6	79.2	82.8	86.4
70	25.2	29.4	33.6	37.8	42	46.2	50.4	54.6	58.8	63	67.2	71.4	75.6	79.8	84	88.2	92.4	96.6	101
80	28.8	33.6	38.4	43.2	48	52.8	57.6	62.4	67.2	72	76.8	81.6	86.4	91.2	96	101	106	110	115
90	32.4	37.8	43.2	48.6	54	59.4	64.8	70.2	75.6	81	86.4	91.8	97.2	103	108	113	119	124	130
100	36	42	48	54	60	66	72	78	84	90	96	102	108	114	120	126	132	138	144

■ Table 60.8 Dobutamine infusion: 500 mg in 50 ml (10 mg/ml)

Infusion volumes (ml/hour)

Dose (µg/kg/min)	Weight (kg) 30	35	40	45	50	55	60	65	70	75	80	85	90	95	100	105	110	115	120
1	0.18	0.21	0.24	0.27	0.3	0.33	0.36	0.39	0.42	0.45	0.48	0.51	0.54	0.57	0.6	0.63	0.66	0.69	0.72
2	0.36	0.42	0.48	0.54	0.6	0.66	0.72	0.78	0.84	0.9	0.96	1.02	1.08	1.14	1.2	1.26	1.32	1.38	1.44
3	0.54	0.63	0.72	0.81	0.9	0.99	1.08	1.17	1.26	1.35	1.44	1.53	1.62	1.71	1.8	1.89	1.98	2.07	2.16
4	0.72	0.84	0.96	1.08	1.2	1.32	1.44	1.56	1.68	1.8	1.92	2.04	2.16	2.28	2.4	2.52	2.64	2.76	2.88
5	0.9	1.05	1.2	1.35	1.5	1.65	1.8	1.95	2.1	2.25	2.4	2.55	2.7	2.85	3	3.15	3.3	3.45	3.6
6	1.08	1.26	1.44	1.62	1.8	1.98	2.16	2.34	2.52	2.7	2.88	3.06	3.24	3.42	3.6	3.78	3.96	4.14	4.32
7	1.26	1.47	1.68	1.89	2.1	2.31	2.52	2.73	2.94	3.15	3.36	3.57	3.78	3.99	4.2	4.41	4.62	4.83	5.04
8	1.44	1.68	1.92	2.16	2.4	2.64	2.88	3.12	3.36	3.6	3.84	4.08	4.32	4.56	4.8	5.04	5.28	5.52	5.76
9	1.62	1.89	2.16	2.43	2.7	2.97	3.24	3.51	3.78	4.05	4.32	4.59	4.86	5.13	5.4	5.67	5.94	6.21	6.48
10	1.8	2.1	2.4	2.7	3	3.3	3.6	3.9	4.2	4.5	4.8	5.1	5.4	5.7	6	6.3	6.6	6.9	7.2
20	3.6	4.2	4.8	5.4	6	6.6	7.2	7.8	8.4	9	9.6	10.2	10.8	11.4	12	12.6	13.2	13.8	14.4

Continued on p. 384

■ Table 60.8 (Continued)

Infusion volumes (ml/hour)

Dose (µg/kg/min)	Weight (kg)																		
	30	35	40	45	50	55	60	65	70	75	80	85	90	95	100	105	110	115	120
30	5.4	6.3	7.2	8.1	9	9.9	10.8	11.7	12.6	13.5	14.4	15.3	16.2	17.1	18	18.9	19.8	20.7	21.6
40	7.2	8.4	9.6	10.8	12	13.2	14.4	15.6	16.8	18	19.2	20.4	21.6	22.8	24	25.2	26.4	27.6	28.8
50	9	10.5	12	13.5	15	16.5	18	19.5	21	22.5	24	25.5	27	28.5	30	31.5	33	34.5	36
60	10.8	12.6	14.4	16.2	18	19.8	21.6	23.4	25.2	27	28.8	30.6	32.4	34.2	36	37.8	39.6	41.4	43.2
70	12.6	14.7	16.8	18.9	21	23.1	25.2	27.3	29.4	31.5	33.6	35.7	37.8	39.9	42	44.1	46.2	48.3	50.4
80	14.4	16.8	19.2	21.6	24	26.4	28.8	31.2	33.6	36	38.4	40.8	43.2	45.6	48	50.4	52.8	55.2	57.6
90	16.2	18.9	21.6	24.3	27	29.7	32.4	35.1	37.8	40.5	43.2	45.9	48.6	51.3	54	56.7	59.4	62.1	64.8
100	18	21	24	27	30	33	36	39	42	45	48	51	54	57	60	63	66	69	72

Dopamine

■ Table 60.9 Dopamine infusion: 2.5 µg/kg/min (renal vasodilator dose)

Infusion volumes (ml/hour)

Concentration	Weight (kg)																		
	30	35	40	45	50	55	60	65	70	75	80	85	90	95	100	105	110	115	120
Dopamine 200 mg in 50 ml	1.1	1.3	1.5	1.7	1.9	2.1	2.3	2.4	2.6	2.8	3	3.2	3.4	3.6	3.8	3.9	4.1	4.3	4.5
Dopamine 400 mg in 50 ml	0.6	0.7	0.8	0.8	0.9	1	1.1	1.2	1.3	1.4	1.5	1.6	1.7	1.8	1.9	2	2.1	2.2	2.3
Dopamine 800 mg in 50 ml	0.3	0.3	0.4	0.4	0.5	0.5	0.6	0.6	0.7	0.7	0.8	0.8	0.8	0.9	0.9	1	1	1.1	1.1

Heparin

■ **Table 60.10** Heparin infusion

Loading dose

5000 U IV over 5 min

Infusion

- 25 000 U made up in saline to 50 ml (500 U/ml)
- Start the infusion at 1400 U/hour (2.8 ml/hour) using a syringe pump
- Check the activated partial thromboplastin time (APTT) at 6 hours
- Adjust the dose as follows:

APTT ratio (target 1.5–2.5)	Change in fusion rate
>7.0	Stop for 30–60 min and reduce dose by 500 U/hour
5.1–7.0	Reduce by 500 U/hour
4.1–5.0	Reduce by 300 U/hour
3.1–4.0	Reduce by 100 U/hour
2.6–3.0	Reduce by 50 U/hour
1.5–2.5	No change
1.2–1.4	Increase by 200 U/hour
<1.2	Increase by 400 U/hour

- After each change in infusion rate, wait 10 hours before next APTT estimation unless APTT ratio is >5.0, in which case check 4-hourly
- Check APTT daily
- Heparin can cause thrombocytopenia: check the platelet count daily if given for longer than 5 days

Reference:
Drug and Therapeutics Bulletin 1992; 30: 77–80.
Adapted from:
Fennerty A *et al.* Anticoagulants in venous thromboembolism. *BMJ* 1988; 297: 1285–8.

Warfarin

Drug interactions with warfarin are common and can be serious. When starting or stopping a treatment, check the list in the *British National Formulary*.

■ **Table 60.11** Indications for warfarin anticoagulation

Indication	Target INR
Prevention of deep-vein thrombosis	2–3
Treatment of deep-vein thrombosis or pulmonary embolism	2–3
Treatment of recurrent deep-vein thrombosis or pulmonary embolism	3–4.5
Atrial fibrillation: prevention of thrombo-embolism	2–3
Acute myocardial infarction: prevention of recurrence and reduction of mortality	3–4.5
Bioprosthetic heart valve	2–3
Mechanical prosthetic heart valve	3–4.5

INR, International Normalized Ratio.
Reference:
Hirsh J. Oral anticoagulant drugs. *N Engl J Med* 1991; 324: 1865–75.

■ **Table 60.12** Clinical conditions affecting response to warfarin

Increased anticoagulation

- Impaired liver function
- Renal failure
- Malabsorptive states
- Congestive heart failure
- Hyperthyroidism

Decreased anticoagulation

- Hypothyroidism
- Transfusion of whole blood or fresh frozen plasma
- Diet high in vitamin K (green vegetables)
- Hereditary resistance to warfarin

■ **Table 60.13** Starting warfarin

Day	INR* (9−11 am)	Warfarin dose (mg) given at 5−7 pm
1	< 1.4	10
	< 1.8	10
2	1.8	1
	> 1.8	0.5
3	< 2.0	10
	2.0−2.1	5
	2.2−2.3	4.5
	2.4−2.5	4
	2.6−2.7	3.5
	2.8−2.9	3
	3.0−3.1	2.5
	3.2−3.3	2
	3.4	1.5
	3.5	1
	3.6−4.0	0.5
	> 4.0	0

		Predicted maintenance dose
4	< 1.4	> 8
	1.4	8
	1.5	7.5
	1.6−1.7	7
	1.8	6.5
	1.9	6
	2.0−2.1	5.5
	2.2−2.3	5
	2.4−2.6	4.5
	2.7−3.0	4
	3.1−3.5	3.5
	3.6−4.0	3
	4.1−4.5	Miss out next day's dose then give 2 mg
	> 4.5	Miss out two days' doses then give 1 mg

INR, International Normalized Ratio; APTT, activated partial thromboplastin time.

* APTT should be within or below therapeutic range (1.5−2.5 × control). If APTT is above this range, the heparin effect on INR should be neutralised by adding protamine (0.4 mcg/ml plasma) to the sample.

Reference:

Drug and Therapeutics Bulletin 1992; 30: 77−80.

Table modified from:

Fennerty A *et al.* Anticoagulants in venous thromboembolism. *BMJ* 1988; 297: 1285−8.

■ **Table 60.14** Management of warfarin overanticoagulation

INR	Clinical condition	Action
4.5–7.0	No bleeding	Stop warfarin for one to two doses
>7.0	No bleeding No prosthetic heart valve	Stop warfarin for one to two doses. Give vitamin K_1 0.5 mg by slow IV injection
	No bleeding Prosthetic heart valve	Stop warfarin for one to two doses. Seek expert advice from a cardiologist*
>1.3	Bleeding or rapid reversal for surgery needed	Stop warfarin. Give vitamin K_1† If full reversal is needed, give prothrombin complex concentrate, 50 U of factor IX per kg, or fresh frozen plasma, 1 l

INR, International Normalized Ratio.
* Full reversal of anticoagulation in patients with mechanical prosthetic heart valves carries a risk of valve thrombosis.
† Give Vitamin K_1 0.5 mg IV if resumption of warfarin anticoagulation is intended. If not, give 5 mg IV by slow injection.

61 ECG and chest X-ray

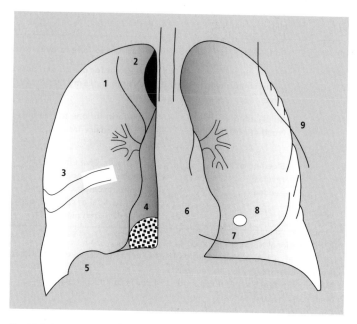

Fig. 61.1 Common normal variants seen on chest X-ray.

1, Azygous lobe (mistaken for bulla or pneumothorax). **2**, Prominant brachio-cephalic vessels (mistaken for upper mediastinal mass or lymphadenopathy). **3**, Calcified costal cartilages (mistaken for pleural or pulmonary lesions). **4**, Peri-cardial cyst or fat pad (mistaken for cardiomegaly, tumour or consolidation). **5**, Diaphragmatic hump (mistaken for tumour or consolidation). **6**, Unusual cardiac shape or apparent cardiomegaly may be caused by pectus excavatum (confirmed by clinical examination). **7**, Asymmetrical breast shadows (mistaken for lower-zone consolidation). **8**, Prominent nipple shadow (mistaken for pulmonary nodule). **9**, Loose folds of skin (especially in anteroposterior supine film). These may be mistaken for a pneumothorax. From O'Driscoll BR, *et al.* ABC of emergency radiology: chest radiographs I. *BMJ* 1993; 1202–6.

Order of appearance while recording

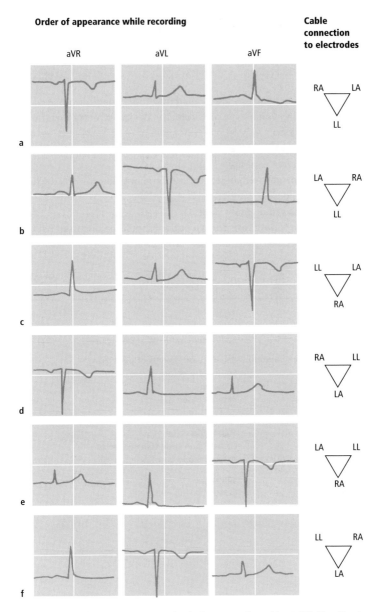

Fig. 61.2 Guide to incorrect ECG lead placement. From Hurst JW. The Heart, Arteries and Veins. 6th edn. New York: McGraw-Hill, 1985; 226.

62 Respiratory function tests

Respiratory-function tests are divided into four broad groups:
- **dynamic lung volumes**, e.g. spirometry, peak expiratory flow rate, flow/volume loop;
- **static lung volumes**, e.g. total lung capacity, residual volume, functional reserve capacity;
- **measures of gas exchange**, e.g. carbon monoxide transfer factor, arterial blood gases;
- **exercise tests**, e.g. 6-min walk.

The most appropriate tests for the patient should be discussed with a chest physician. For guidelines, see Table 62.1.

■ **Table 62.1** Choosing respiratory-function tests

Condition	Tests
Asthma	Serial measurements of peak flow
Chronic airflow limitation	Serial measurements of peak flow
	Spirometry before and after bronchodilator therapy
	Arterial blood gases
Interstitial lung disease	Spirometry
	Static lung volumes
	Carbon monoxide transfer factor
	Arterial blood gases
Preoperative assessment	Spirometry
	Exercise test (6-min walk)
Extrathoracic airways obstruction	Flow/volume loop

■ **Table 62.2** Peak expiratory flow rate in males (l/min)

Height (ft/inches)	Age (years) 20–25	30	35	40	45	50	55	60	65	70
5'3"	572	560	548	536	524	512	500	488	476	464
5'6"	597	584	572	559	547	534	522	509	496	484
5'9"	625	612	599	586	573	560	547	533	520	507
6'0"	654	640	626	613	599	585	572	558	544	530
6'3"	679	665	650	636	622	608	593	579	565	551

Standard deviation 60 l/min.

■ **Table 62.3** Peak expiratory flow rate in females (l/min)

Height (ft/inches)	Age (years) 20–25	30	35	40	45	50	55	60	65	70
4'9"	377	366	356	345	335	324	314	303	293	282
5'0"	403	392	382	371	361	350	340	329	319	308
5'3"	433	422	412	401	391	380	370	359	349	338
5'6"	459	448	438	427	417	406	396	385	375	364
5'9"	489	478	468	457	447	436	426	415	405	394

Standard deviation 60 l/min.

■ **Table 62.4** Forced expiratory volume in 1 s (FEV_1) in males (l)

Height (ft/inches)	Age (years) 20–25	30	35	40	45	50	55	60	65	70
5'3"	3.61	3.45	3.30	3.14	2.99	2.83	2.68	2.52	2.37	2.21
5'6"	3.86	3.71	3.55	3.40	3.24	3.09	2.93	2.78	2.62	2.47
5'9"	4.15	4.00	3.84	3.69	3.53	3.38	3.22	3.06	2.91	2.75
6'0"	4.44	4.28	4.13	3.97	3.82	3.66	3.51	3.35	3.20	3.04
6'3"	4.69	4.54	4.38	4.23	4.07	3.92	3.76	3.61	3.45	3.30

Standard deviation 0.5 l.

■ **Table 62.5** Forced expiratory volume in 1 s in females (l)

Height (ft/inches)	Age (years) 20–25	30	35	40	45	50	55	60	65	70
4'9"	2.60	2.45	2.30	2.15	2.00	1.85	1.70	1.55	1.40	1.25
5'0"	2.83	2.68	2.53	2.38	2.23	2.08	1.93	1.78	1.63	1.48
5'3"	3.09	2.94	2.79	2.64	2.49	2.34	2.19	2.04	1.89	1.74
5'6"	3.36	3.21	3.06	2.91	2.76	2.61	2.46	2.31	2.16	2.01
5'9"	3.59	3.44	3.29	3.14	2.99	2.84	2.69	2.54	2.39	2.24

Standard deviation 0.4 l.

■ **Table 62.6** Forced vital capacity in males (l)

Height (ft/inches)	Age (years) 20–25	30	35	40	45	50	55	60	65	70
5'3"	4.17	4.06	3.95	3.84	3.73	3.62	3.51	3.40	3.29	3.18
5'6"	4.53	4.42	4.31	4.20	4.09	3.98	3.87	3.76	3.65	3.54
5'9"	4.95	4.84	4.73	4.62	4.51	4.40	4.29	4.18	4.07	3.96
6'0"	5.37	5.26	5.15	5.04	4.93	4.82	4.71	4.60	4.49	4.38
6'3"	5.73	5.62	5.51	5.40	5.29	5.18	5.07	4.96	4.85	4.74

Standard deviation 0.6 l.

■ **Table 62.7** Forced vital capacity in females (l)

Height (ft/inches)	Age (years) 20–25	30	35	40	45	50	55	60	65	70
4'9"	3.13	2.98	2.83	2.68	2.53	2.38	2.23	2.08	1.93	1.78
5'0"	3.45	3.30	3.15	3.00	2.85	2.70	2.55	2.40	2.25	2.10
5'3"	3.83	3.68	3.53	3.38	3.23	3.08	2.93	2.78	2.63	2.48
5'6"	4.20	4.05	3.90	3.75	3.60	3.45	3.30	3.15	3.00	2.85
5'9"	4.53	4.38	4.23	4.08	3.93	3.78	3.63	3.48	3.33	3.18

Standard deviation 0.4 l.

■ **Table 62.8** FEV_1 as a percentage of forced vital capacity (%)

	Age (years)									
	20–25	30	35	40	45	50	55	60	65	70
Males*	82.5	80.6	78.7	76.9	75.0	73.1	71.3	69.4	67.5	65.7
Females†	81.0	79.9	78.8	77.7	76.6	75.5	74.3	73.2	72.1	71.0

* Standard deviation 7%.

† Standard deviation 6%.

Notes on Tables 62.2−62.8

● The mean ± one standard deviation includes 68% of healthy subjects; 2 standard deviations include 95% of healthy subjects.

● FEV_1 and FVC: the values shown are for people of European descent; for races with smaller thoraces (e.g. from the Indian subcontinent and Polynesia), subtract 0.4 l from the values given for FEV_1 and 0.7 l for FVC in males and 0.6 l in females.

Reference:

Cotes JE. *Lung Function.* 4th edn. Oxford: Blackwell Scientific Publications, 1978.

63 Arterial blood gases and pH

Arterial blood sampling

1 Always wear gloves for your own protection.

2 Samples can be taken from the radial or brachial artery. If you use the brachial artery, the elbow should be fully extended over a pillow to prevent movement of the artery during sampling.

3 Inject 1 ml of lignocaine into the skin and around the artery: pain leads to hyperventilation.

4 Locate the artery with two fingers to establish its course and advance the needle into the segment between your fingers.

5 The needle should be angled at about 45°. Sampling 2 ml of blood is usually sufficient.

6 After removing the needle, put direct pressure on the artery using a folded gauze swab.

7 If sampling from the brachial artery, an elasticated crepe bandage should be wound tightly round the elbow: instruct the patient to call for it to be removed in 5 min in case it is forgotten. If the radial is being used apply direct pressure for 5 min: do not leave this for the patient to do themselves as firm pressure is needed to prevent bruising, and bruising around the radial artery can be very painful for several hours or days.

8 Expel any small bubbles from the syringe immediately.

9 Remove the needle directly into a disposal bin and cap the syringe.

10 Analyse immediately or place in a mixture of ice and water – ice alone may lead to haemolysis.

11 Check for bleeding and apply a plaster.

Reference values

1 Normal values:
- **pHa**   7.35–7.45 (35–45 nmol/l)

■ **Table 63.1** Hydrogen ion concentration: conversion of pH units to nmol/l

	Hydrogen ion concentration (nmol/l)									
pH	0	1	2	3	4	5	6	7	8	9
7.0	99	97	95	93	91	89	87	85	83	81
7.1	79	78	76	74	72	71	69	68	66	65
7.2	63	62	60	59	58	56	55	54	53	51
7.3	50	49	48	47	46	45	44	43	42	41
7.4	40	39	38	37	36	35	35	34	33	32
7.5	31	30	30	30	29	28	28	27	26	26
7.6	25	25	24	23	23	22	22	21	21	20

- Pa_{O_2} 10.0–13.3 kPa (75–100 mmHg)
- Pa_{CO_2} 4.7–6.0 kPa (35–45 mmHg)

2 Respiratory failure is defined as a $Pa_{O_2} < 8$ kPa or $Pa_{CO_2} > 7$ kPa, breathing air.

3 Conversion factors.
- pH units to nmol/l: see Table 63.1.
- kPa to mmHg: multiply by 7.5.
- mmHg to kPa: divide by 0.133.

4 Correction of Pa_{O_2} for age:
predicted normal value (mmHg) = 104 − (age (years) × 0.27)

5 Correction for body temperature: see Table 63.2.

■ **Table 63.2** Correction of arterial pH and blood gases for body temperature

	Change of body temperature from 37°C	
	Increase 1°C	Decrease 1°C
pHa	Down 0.015	Up 0.015
Pa_{O_2}	Up 4.4%	Down 4.4%
Pa_{CO_2}	Up 7.2%	Down 7.2%

References:

Normal reference values. *N Engl J Med* 1986; 314: 39–49.

Mellemgaard K. The alveolar-arterial oxygen difference: its size and components in normal man. *Acta Physiol Scand* 1966; 67: 16–20.

Reuler JB. Hypothermia: pathophysiology, clinical settings, and management. *Ann Intern Med* 1978; 89: 519–27.

Interpretation of results

Always look at (and record) the inspired oxygen concentration along with the Po_2 – a normal Po_2 on supplemental oxygen is in fact abnormal!

- A normal Po_2 may be maintained by hyperventilation.
- Arterial $Po_2 < 8\,kPa$ (60 mmHg) indicates respiratory failure.

The absolute value of arterial Pco_2 is of less significance than the arterial Pco_2/pH relationship.

■ **Table 63.3** Causes of an acute metabolic acidosis

---

1 Lactic acidosis
  - Inadequate tissue perfusion due to hypotension, low cardiac output or sepsis
  - Prolonged hypoxaemia
  - Muscle contraction: status epilepticus
2 Diabetic ketoacidosis (p. 253)
3 Alcoholic ketoacidosis*
4 Acute renal failure (p. 238)
5 Poisoning
  - Carbon monoxide (p. 103)
  - Ethanol
  - Ethylene glycol
  - Methanol
  - Paracetamol (p. 99)
  - Salicylates (p. 99)
  - Tricyclics

---

* Due to alcohol binge plus starvation; often associated with pancreatitis; hyperglycaemia may occur but is mild (< 15 mmol/l); treat with IV dextrose infusion; other supportive therapy is given on p. 70.

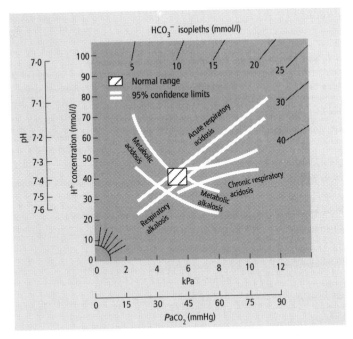

Fig. 63.1 Acid–base diagram relating arterial hydrogen ion concentration (nmol/l) to P_{aCO_2} within the body. The shaded rectangle is the normal range. The 95% confidence limits of hydrogen ion concentration/P_{aCO_2} relationships in single disturbances of acid–base balance are shown. From Flenley DC. Another non-logarithmic acid-base diagram? *Lancet* 1971; 1: 961, © by The Lancet Ltd.

- Compare the P_{CO_2} and pH (or plot the P_{CO_2} against pH on the nomogram; see Fig. 63.1) to establish the acid–base status.
- Remember that prolonged hypoxaemia is a cause of metabolic acidosis. Other causes are given in Table 63.3.
- Only look at the base excess to confirm your diagnosis.

64 Peripheral nervous system

■ Table 64.1 Muscle groups: root and peripheral nerve supply

Movement	Muscle group	Main roots	Peripheral nerve
Shoulder abduction	Deltoid	C5	Axillary
Shoulder adduction	Latissimus dorsi	C7	Brachial plexus
	Pectoralis major	C5–7	Brachial plexus
Elbow flexion	Biceps	C5–6	Musculocutaneous
	Brachioradialis	C6	Radial
Elbow extension	Triceps	C7	Radial
Wrist flexion	Flexor muscles of forearm	C7–8	Median/ulnar
Wrist extension	Extensor muscles of forearm	C7	Radial
Finger flexion	Flexor muscles of forearm	C7–8	Median/ulnar
Finger extension	Extensor muscles of forearm	C7	Radial
Finger abduction	Interossei	T1	Ulnar
	Abductor digiti minimi	T1	Ulnar
Thumb abduction	Abductor pollicis brevis	T1	Median
Hip flexion	Iliopsoas	L1–2	Femoral
Hip extension	Gluteus maximus	L5–S1	Inferior gluteal
Hip abduction	Gluteus medius and minimus	L4–5	Superior gluteal
	Tensor fasciae latae	L4–5	Superior gluteal
Hip adduction	Adductors	L2–3	Obturator

Continued

■ Table **64.1** *(Continued)*

Movement	Muscle group	Main roots	Peripheral nerve
Knee flexion	Hamstrings	S1	Sciatic
Knee extension	Quadriceps	L3–4	Femoral
Ankle dorsiflexion	Tibialis anterior	L4	Sciatic (peroneal)
Ankle plantarflexion	Gastrocnemius	S1–2	Sciatic (tibial)
Ankle eversion	Peroneus longus	L5–S1	Sciatic (peroneal)
Ankle inversion	Tibialis anterior	L4	Sciatic (peroneal)
	Tibialis posterior	L4–5	Sciatic (tibial)
Great-toe dorsiflexion	Extensor hallucis longus	L5	Sciatic (peroneal)

Reference:
Medical Research Council Memorandum No. 45. Aids to the examination of the peripheral nervous system. London: Her Majesty's Stationery Office, 1976.

■ Table **64.2** Tendon reflexes: root and peripheral nerve supply

Tendon reflex	Muscle	Main roots	Peripheral nerve
Biceps	Biceps	C5–6	Musculocutaneous
Supinator	Brachioradialis	C6	Radial
Triceps	Triceps	C7	Radial
Finger	Long finger flexors	C7–8	Median/ulnar
Knee	Quadriceps	L3–4	Femoral
Ankle	Gastrocnemius	S1–2	Sciatic (tibial)

Reference:
Medical Research Council Memorandum No. 45. Aids to the examination of the peripheral nervous system. London: Her Majesty's Stationery Office, 1976.

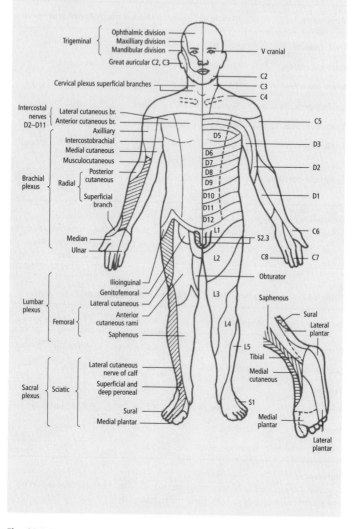

Fig. 64.1 Sensory innervation of the skin. Cutaneous areas of distribution of spinal segments and sensory fibres of the peripheral nerves: anterior and

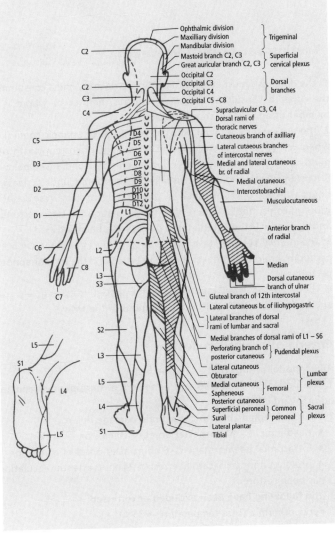

Ophthalmic division
Maxilliary division } Trigeminal
Mandibular division

Mastoid branch C2, C3 } Superficial
Great auricular branch C2, C3 } cervical plexus

Occipital C2
Occipital C3 } Dorsal
Occipital C4 } branches
Occipital C5 –C8

Supraclavicular C3, C4
Dorsal rami of thoracic nerves
Cutaneous branch of axilliary
Lateral cutaeous branches of intercostal nerves
Medial and lateral cutaneous br. of radial
Medial cutaneous
Intercostobrachial
Musculocutaneous

Anterior branch of radial

Median
Dorsal cutaneous branch of ulnar
Gluteal branch of 12th intercostal
Lateral cutaneous br. of iliohypogastric
Lateral branches of dorsal rami of lumbar and sacral
Medial branches of dorsal rami of L1 – S6
Perforating branch of posterior cutaneous } Pudendal plexus
Lateral cutaneous
Obturator } Lumbar
Medial cutaneous } Femoral } plexus
Sapheneous
Posterior cutaneous
Superficial peroneal } Common } Sacral
Sural } peroneal } plexus
Lateral plantar
Tibial

Fig. 64.1 *(Continued)* posterior views. From *Brain's Diseases of the Nervous System*. 10th edn. Oxford: Oxford University Press, 1993.

65 Brainstem death

Testing for brainstem death

1 The diagnosis must be confirmed by two doctors, one a consultant, the other a consultant or senior registrar, neither of whom is a member of an organ transplant team.

2 The appropriate interval between the onset of apnoeic coma (i.e. when ventilation was started) and testing for brainstem death depends on the time required to establish criteria 2 and 3 (see below). Brainstem death should not usually be considered until at least 6 hours after the onset of coma, or, if anoxia or cardiac arrest was the cause of coma, until 24 hours after the circulation has been restored, and then only if the criteria listed below have been satisfied.

3 The interval between tests should be 2–3 hours or longer. On both occasions, brainstem reflexes should be tested and the test for apnoea performed.

4 There are no legal requirements for special tests (e.g. electro-encephalography) to confirm the diagnosis in the UK.

Criteria of brainstem death

All of the following criteria must be met.

1 **The patient is comatose and apnoeic** (i.e. unresponsive and requiring ventilation).

2 **There is irremediable structural brain damage due to:**
- head injury (>6 hours after onset of coma); or
- intracranial haemorrhage (>6 hours after onset of coma); or
- prolonged anoxia or cardiac arrest (>24 hours after the circulation has been restored).

3 **The following have been excluded or corrected:**
- hypothermia (core temperature $>35°C$);
- drug or alcohol intoxication;
- metabolic or endocrine derangement (where appropriate check plasma sodium, glucose and calcium);

- neuromuscular blockade (no neuromuscular blocking drugs administered during the preceding 12 hours).

4 There are no brainstem reflexes.

5 The patient remains apnoeic on disconnection from the ventilator.

Testing of brainstem reflexes and for apnoea

The following reflexes must all be tested.

1 Pupillary response to light.
- A bright light must be used.
- Atropine (pupil dilated) and neuromuscular blockers (pupil midposition) can abolish the response.

2 Corneal reflex.
- Apply firm pressure on the cornea using a sterile swab.
- Observe for blinking of either eye.

3 Oculocephalic reflex.
- Rotate the head fully to left and right.
- If the brainstem is intact, both eyes conjugately rotate counter to the movement of the head.

4 Vestibulo-ocular reflex.
- Both sides should be tested in turn.
- Use an auriscope to check the ear canal is free of wax. If wax is blocking the ear canal it must be removed.
- Irrigate with 50 ml of ice-cold water for 30 s: the tubing of a 'Butterfly' needle (with the needle cut off) can be used.
- Observe for movement of either eye: any movement signifies brainstem activity.

5 Cranial motor response to somatic stimulation.
- Apply firm supra-orbital and nailbed pressure.
- Observe for grimacing.

6 Reflex response to bronchial stimulation.
- Pass a suction catheter down the endotracheal tube into the trachea and bronchi.
- Observe for coughing or gagging.

7 Test for apnoea.

- Pre-oxygenate the patient by ventilating for 10 min with 100% oxygen.

- Check blood gases. $Pa{CO_2}$ before disconnection must be > 5.3 kPa (40 mmHg); if lower than this, reduce the frequency of ventilation or ventilate with 5% carbon dioxide in 95% oxygen for 5 min and recheck.

- Disconnect the patient from the ventilator. Maintain oxygenation during disconnection by placing a catheter in the trachea with an oxygen flow rate of 6 l/min.

- Observe for respiratory efforts.

- Recheck gases after 10 min: $Pa{CO_2}$ must be > 6.7 kPa (50 mmHg) to confirm an adequate test.

Further reading

1 Cardiac arrest

European Resuscitation Council Working Party. Guidelines for Basic Life Support. *BMJ* 1993; 306: 1587–9.

European Resuscitation Council Working Party. Guidelines for Advanced Cardiac Life Support. *BMJ* 1993; 306: 1589–93.

O'Nunain S, Ruskin J. Cardiac arrest. *Lancet* 1993; 341: 1641–7.

2 Cardiac arrhythmias

Murgatroyd FD, Camm AJ. Atrial arrhythmias. *Lancet* 1993; 341: 1317–22.

Kuck K-H, Schluter M. Junctional tachycardia and the role of catheter ablation. *Lancet* 1993; 341: 1386–91.

Campbell RWF. Ventricular ectopic beats and non-sustained ventricular tachycardia. *Lancet* 1993; 341: 1454–8.

Shenasa M, *et al*. Ventricular tachycardia. *Lancet* 1993; 341: 1512–19.

Ben-David J, Zipes DP. Torsades de pointes and proarrhythmia. *Lancet* 1993; 341: 1578–82.

3 Hypotension

Bradley RD. *Studies in Acute Heart Failure*. London: Edward Arnold, 1977.

Shoemaker WC, *et al*. Oxygen transport measurements to evaluate tissue perfusion and titrate therapy: dobutamine and dopamine effects. *Crit Care Med* 1991; 19: 672–88.

Fiddian-Green RC, *et al*. Goals for the resuscitation of shock. *Crit Care Med* 1993; 21 (suppl): S25–31.

4 Acute chest pain

Lee TH, *et al*. Ruling out acute myocardial infarction – a prospective multicenter validation of a 12-hour strategy for patients at low risk. *N Engl J Med* 1991; 324: 1239–46.

Rude RE, *et al*. Electrocardiographic and clinical criteria for recognition of acute myocardial infarction based on analysis of 3,697 patients. *Am J Cardiol* 1983; 52: 936–42.

Henderson JAM, Peloquin AJM. Boerhaave revisited: spontaneous esophageal perforation as a diagnostic masquerader. *Am J Med* 1989; 86: 559–67.

Aase O, *et al*. Decision support by computer analysis of selected case history variables in the emergency room among patients with acute chest pain. *Eur Heart J* 1993; 14: 433–40.

5 Acute breathlessness

Howell JBL. Behavioural breathlessness. *Thorax* 1990; 45: 287–92.

6 The unconscious patient

Plum F, Posner JB. *The Diagnosis of Stupor and Coma.* 3rd edn. Philadelphia: FA Davis company, 1980.

7 Transient loss of consciousness

Petch M. Syncope. *BMJ* 1994; 308: 1251–2.

Manolis AS, *et al.* Syncope: current diagnostic evaluation and management. *Ann Intern Med* 1990; 112: 850–63.

Kapoor WN. Evaluation and outcome of patients with syncope. *Medicine* (Baltimore) 1990; 69: 160–75.

8 Acute confusional state

Charness ME, *et al.* Ethanol and the nervous system. *N Engl J Med* 1989; 321: 442–54.

Editorial. Non-convulsive status epilepticus. *Lancet* 1987; 1: 958–9.

Lipowski ZJ. Current concepts: Delirium in the elderly patient. *N Engl J Med* 1989; 320: 578–82.

9 Headache

Lance JW. Treatment of migraine. *Lancet* 1992; 339: 1207–9.

Ostergaard JR. Warning leak in subarachnoid haemmorhage. *BMJ* 1990; 301: 190–1.

Clough C. Non-migrainous headaches. *BMJ* 1989; 299: 70–2.

10 Sepsis and sepsis syndrome

Glauser MP, *et al.* Septic shock: pathogenesis. *Lancet* 1991; 338: 732–6.

Cohen J, Glauser MP. Septic shock: treatment. *Lancet* 1991; 338: 736–9.

Parrillo JE. Mechanisms of disease: Pathogenetic mechanisms of septic shock. *N Engl J Med* 1993; 328: 1471–7.

Edwards JD. Management of septic shock. *BMJ* 1993; 306: 1661–4.

11 Poisoning

Kulig K. Current concepts: Initial management of ingestion of toxic substances. *N Engl J Med* 1992; 326: 1677–81.

12 Acute myocardial infarction

ACC/AHA guidelines for the early management of patients with acute myocardial infarction. *Circulation* 1990; 82: 664–707.

Weston CFM, *et al.* Guidelines for the early management of patients with myocardial infarction. *BMJ* 1994; 308: 767–71.

Anderson HV, Willerson JT. Current concepts: Thrombolysis in acute myocardial infarction. *N Engl J Med* 1993; 329: 703–9.

Kinch JW, Ryan TJ. Current concepts: Right ventricular infarction. *N Engl J Med* 1994; 330: 1211–17.

Vannan MA, *et al.* ACE inhibitors after myocardial infarction. *BMJ* 1993; 306: 531–2.

13 Unstable angina

Theroux P, *et al.* Reactivation of unstable angina after the discontinuation of heparin. *N Engl J Med* 1992; 327: 141–5.

Casscells W, *et al.* Thrombus and unstable angina. *Lancet* 1993; 342: 1151–5.

Bar FW, *et al.* Thrombolysis in patients with unstable angina improves the angiographic but not the clinical outcome. *Circulation* 1992; 86: 131–7.

14 Aortic dissection

Treasure T, Raphael MJ. Investigation of suspected dissection of the thoracic aorta. *Lancet* 1991; 338: 490–5.

Cigarroa JE, *et al.* Diagnostic imaging in the evaluation of suspected aortic dissection – old standards and new directions. *N Engl J Med* 1993; 328: 35–43.

15 Severe hypertension

Calhoun DA, Oparil S. Current concepts: Treatment of hypertensive crisis. *N Engl J Med* 1990; 323: 1177–83.

Kincaid-Smith P. Malignant hypertension. *J Hypertens* 1991; 9: 893–9.

16 Pulmonary oedema

Bersten AD, *et al.* Treatment of severe cardiogenic pulmonary edema with continuous positive airway pressure delivered by face mask. *N Engl J Med* 1991; 325: 1825–30.

Macnaughton PD, Evans TW. Management of adult respiratory distress syndrome. *Lancet* 1992; 339: 469–72.

Tobin MJ. Current concepts: Mechanical ventilation. *N Engl J Med* 1994; 330: 1056–61.

17 Pericarditis

Spodick DH. The normal and diseased pericardium: Current concepts of pericardial physiology, diagnosis, and treatment. *J Am Coll Cardiol* 1983; 1: 240.

Corey GR, *et al.* Etiology of large pericardial effusions. *Am J Med* 1993; 95: 209–13.

18 Cardiac tamponade

Guberman BA, *et al.* Cardiac tamponade in medical patients. *Circulation* 1981; 64: 633–40.

Fowler NO. Cardiac tamponade: a clinical or an echocardiographic diagnosis? *Circulation* 1993; 87: 1738–41.

19 Deep-vein thrombosis

Moser KM. State of the art: Venous thromboembolism. *Am Rev Respir Dis* 1990; 141: 235–49.

Hull RD, *et al.* Heparin for 5 days as compared with 10 days in the initial treatment of proximal venous thrombosis. *N Engl J Med* 1990; 322: 1260–4.

Research Committee of the British Thoracic Society. Optimum duration of anticoagulation for deep-vein thrombosis and pulmonary embolism. *Lancet* 1992; 340: 873–6.

20 Pulmonary embolism

PIOPED investigators. Value of the ventilation/perfusion scan in acute pumonary embolism. Results of the prospective investigation of pulmonary embolism diagnosis (PIOPED). *JAMA* 1990; 263: 2753–9.

Morrell NW, Seed WA. Diagnosing pulmonary embolism. *BMJ* 1992; 304: 1126–7.

ten Cate JW. Thrombolytic treatment of pulmonary embolism. *Lancet* 1993; 341: 1315–16.

21 Acute asthma

British Thoracic Society, British Paediatric Association, Royal College of Physicians, Kings Fund Centre, National Asthma Campaign, Royal College of General Practitioners Guidelines on the management of asthma. *Thorax* 1993; 48: S1–24.

Tattersfield AE. Asthma – where now? In: Lawson DH, ed. *Current Medicine* 4. Edinburgh: Churchill Livingstone, 1994; 29–49.

22 Acute exacerbation of chronic airflow limitation

Jeffrey AA, *et al.* Acute hypercapnic respiratory failure in patients with chronic obstructive lung disease: risk factors and guidelines for management. *Thorax* 1992; 470: 34–40.

Murphy TF, Sethi S. State of the art: Bacterial infection in chronic obstructive pulmonary disease. *Am Rev Respir Dis* 1992; 146: 1067–83.

Gribbin HR. Management of respiratory failure. *Br J Hosp Med* 1993; 49: 461–77.

23 Pneumonia

British Thoracic Society Guidelines for the management of community acquired pneumonia in adults admitted to hospital. *Br J Hosp Med* 1993; 49: 346–50.

Hosker HSR, *et al.* Management of community acquired lower respiratory tract infection. *BMJ* 1994; 308: 701–5.

24 Pneumothorax
Miller AC, Harvey JE. Guidelines for the management of spontaneous pneumothorax. *BMJ* 1993; 307: 114–16.

25 Hyperventilation
Howell JBL. Behavioural breathlessness. *Thorax* 1990; 45: 287–92.

26 Haemoptysis
Editorial. Life-threatening haemoptysis. *Lancet* 1987; 1: 1354–6.

27 Stroke
Bamford J, *et al.* Classification and natural history of clinically identifiable subtypes of cerebral infarction. *Lancet* 1991; 337: 1521–6.
Caplan LR. Intracerebral haemorrhage. *Lancet* 1992; 339: 656–8.
Hart RG. Cardiogenic embolism to the brain. *Lancet* 1992; 339: 589–94.
Sandercock PA, Willems H. Medical treatment of acute ischaemic stroke. *Lancet* 1992; 339: 537–9.
Oppenheimer S, Hachinskie V. Complications of acute stroke. *Lancet* 1992; 339: 721–4.
Warlow C. Secondary prevention of stroke. *Lancet* 1992; 339: 724–7.

28 Transient ischaemic attack
Landi G. Clinical diagnosis of transient ischaemic attacks. *Lancet* 1992; 339: 402–5.
Donnan GA. Investigation of patients with stroke and transient ischaemic attacks. *Lancet* 1992; 339: 473–7.
Brown MM, Humphrey PRD. Carotid endarterectomy: recommendations for the management of transient ischaemic attack and ischaemic stroke. *BMJ* 1992; 305: 1071–4.

29 Subarachnoid haemorrhage
van Gijn J. Subarachnoid haemmorhage. *Lancet* 1992; 339: 653–5.

30 Bacterial meningitis
Tunkel AR, *et al.* Bacterial meningitis: Recent advances in pathophysiology and treatment. *Ann Intern Med* 1990; 112: 610–23.
Quagliarello V, Scheld WM. Mechanisms of disease: Bacterial meningitis: pathogenesis, pathophysiology and progress. *N Engl J Med* 1992; 327: 864–72.
Durand ML, *et al.* Acute bacterial meningitis in adults. *N Engl J Med* 1993; 328: 21–8.

31 Spinal cord compression

Byrne TN. Current concepts: Spinal cord compression from epidural metastases. *N Engl J Med* 1992; 327: 614–19.

32 Guillain–Barré syndrome

Ropper AH. Current concepts: The Guillain–Barré syndrome. *N Engl J Med* 1992; 326: 1130–6.

33 Major epilepsy

Scheuer ML, Pedley TA. Current concepts: The evaluation and treatment of seizures. *N Engl J Med* 1990; 323: 1468–73.

Brodie MJ. Status epilepticus in adults. *Lancet* 1990; 336: 551–2.

34 Acute upper gastrointestinal haemorrhage

Joint Working Group Guidelines for good practice in and audit of the management of upper gastrointestinal haemorrhage. *J Roy Coll Phys Lond* 1992; 26: 281–9.

Jones DJ. Lower gastrointestinal haemorrhage. *BMJ* 1992; 305: 107–10.

Williams SGJ, Westaby D. Management of variceal haemorrhage. *BMJ* 1994; 308: 1213–17.

35 Acute hepatic encephalopathy

Lee WM. Acute liver failure. *N Engl J Med* 1993; 329: 1862–72.

36 Acute renal failure

Rose BD. *Pathophysiology of Renal Disease.* 3rd edn. New York: McGraw-Hill, 1992.

37–40 Diabetes

Watkins PJ, *et al. Diabetes and its Management.* 4th edn. Oxford: Blackwell Scientific Publications, 1990.

Hepburn DA, Frier BM. Hypoglycaemia and diabetes. In: Lawson DH, ed. *Current Medicine 4.* Edinburgh: Churchill Livingstone, 1994; 97–120.

Milaskiewicz RM, Hall GM. Diabetes and anaesthesia: the past decade. *Br J Anaes* 1992; 68: 198–206.

41 Hyponatraemia

Cluitmans FHM, Meinders AE. Management of severe hyponatraemia: rapid or slow correction? *Am J Med* 1990; 88: 161–6.

Arieff AI. Management of hyponatraemia. *BMJ* 1993; 307: 305–8.

42 Hypercalcaemia

Bilezikian JP. Management of acute hypercalcaemia. *N Engl J Med* 1992; 326: 1196–203.

Editorial. Treating cancer-associated hypercalcaemia. *Drug Ther Bull* 1990; 28: 85–7.

43 Acute adrenal insufficiency

Clayton RN. Diagnosis of acute adrenal insufficiency. *BMJ* 1989; 298: 271–2.

44 Thyrotoxic Crisis

Burger AG, Philippe J. Thyroid storm. *Clin Endocrinol Metab* 1992; 6: 77–93.

45 Hypothermia and myxoedema coma

Reuler JB. Hypothermia: pathophysiology, clinical settings and management. *Ann Intern Med* 1978; 89: 519–27.

Weinberg AD. Hypothermia. *Ann Emerg Med* 1993; 22: 370–7.

46 Acute medical problems in the patient with HIV/AIDS

Miller RF, Mitchell DM. Pneumocystis carinii pneumonia. *Thorax* 1992; 47: 305–14.

Mitchell DM, Miller RF. Recent developments in the management of pulmonary complications of HIV disease. *Thorax* 1992; 47: 381–90.

Shelhamer JH, *et al.* Respiratory disease in the immunosuppressed patient. *Ann Intern Med* 1992; 117: 415–31.

Wachter RM, *et al.* Critical care of patients with AIDS. *JAMA* 1992; 267: 541–7.

Smith PD, *et al.* Gastrointestinal infections in AIDS. *Ann Intern Med* 1992; 116: 63–77.

47 Septic arthritis

Baker DG, Schumacher HR Jr. Current concepts: Acute monoarthritis. *N Engl J Med* 1993; 329: 1013–20.

48 Anaphylactic shock

Bochner BS, Lichtenstein LM. Anaphylaxis. *N Engl J Med* 1991; 324: 1785–90.

Fisher M. Treating anaphylaxis with sympathomimetic drugs. *BMJ* 1992; 305: 1107–8.

49 Sickle-cell disease

Davies SC. The vaso-occlusive crisis of sickle cell disease. *BMJ* 1991; 302: 1551–2.

Rucknagel DL, *et al.* Rib infarcts and acute chest syndrome in sickle cell diseases. *Lancet* 1991; 337: 831–3.

50 Fever on return from abroad

Molyneux M, Fox R. Diagnosis and treatment of malaria in Britain. *BMJ* 1993; 306: 1175–80.

51 Central vein cannulation

Rosen M, *et al. Handbook of Percutaneous Central Venous Catheterisation.* 2nd edn. London: WB Saunders, 1993.

52 Pulmonary artery catheterization

O'Quin R, Marini JJ. Pulmonary artery occlusion pressure: clinical physiology, measurement and interpretation. *Am Rev Respir Dis* 1983; 128: 319–26.

McGrath RB. Invasive bedside hemodynamic monitoring. *Progr Cardiovasc Dis* 1986; 29: 129–44.

Iberti TJ, *et al.* A multicenter study of physicians' knowledge of the pulmonary artery catheter. *JAMA* 1990; 264: 2928–32.

53 Temporary cardiac pacing

Gulotta SJ. Transvenous cardiac pacing. Technics for optimal electrode positioning and prevention of coronary sinus placement. *Circulation* 1970; 42: 701–18.

Lumia FJ, Rios JC. Temporary transvenous pacemaker therapy: an analysis of complications. *Chest* 1973; 64: 604–8.

54 Pericardial aspiration

Krikorian JG, Hancock EW. Pericardiocentesis. *Am J Med* 1978; 65: 808–14.

Callahan JA, *et al.* Two-dimensional echocardiographically guided pericardiocentesis: experience in 117 consecutive patients. *Am J Cardiol* 1985; 55: 476–9.

55 DC countershock

DeSilva RA, *et al.* Cardioversion and defibrillation. *Am Heart J* 1980; 100: 881–95.

AHA/ACC/ACP Task Force Statement. Clinical competence in elective direct current cardioversion. *Circulation* 1993; 88: 342–5.

56 Insertion of chest drain

Miller KS, Sahn SA. Chest tubes: indications, technique, management and complications. *Chest* 1987; 91: 258–64.

57 Lumbar puncture

Petito F, Plum F. The lumbar puncture. *N Engl J Med* 1974; 290: 225–7.

Pearce JMS. Hazards of lumbar puncture. *BMJ* 1982; 285: 1521–2.

58 Peritoneal dialysis

Miller RB, Tassistro CR. Current concepts: Peritoneal dialysis. *N Engl J Med* 1969; 281: 945–9.

59 Insertion of a Senstaken–Blakemore tube

Vlavianos P, *et al.* Balloon tamponade in variceal bleeding: use and misuse. *BMJ* 1989; 298: 1158.

Index